Ulcerative Colitis - Etiology, Diagnosis, Diet, Special Populations, and the Role of Interventional Endoscopy

Edited by Partha Pal

Published in London, United Kingdom

Ulcerative Colitis - Etiology, Diagnosis, Diet, Special Populations, and the Role of Interventional Endoscopy
http://dx.doi.org/10.5772/intechopen.98065
Edited by Partha Pal

Contributors
Sabina Wiecek, Stanko Petrovic, Slobodan Obradovic, Marijana Petrovic, Nemanja Rancic, Jera Jeruc, Athula Kaluarachchi, Nilesh Fernandopulle, Probhodana Ranaweera, Dinindu Kaluarachchi, Indumini Kaluarachchi, Sanupa Kumarasiri Jayawardena, Gayana Mahendra, Janaki Hewavisenthi, Md. Alauddin, Abul Fazal Mohammad Nazmus Sadat, Afroza Sultana, Rayna Shentova-Eneva, Ivan Yankov, Carmen-Monica Preda, Doina Istrătescu, Partha Pal, Mohan Ramchandani, Rupa Banerjee, Duvvuru Nageshwar Reddy, Manu Tandan, Zaheer Nabi

First published in London, United Kingdom, 2022 by IntechOpen
IntechOpen is the global imprint of INTECHOPEN LIMITED, registered in England and Wales, registration number: 11086078, 5 Princes Gate Court, London, SW7 2QJ, United Kingdom

British Library Cataloguing-in-Publication Data
A catalogue record for this book is available from the British Library

Additional hard and PDF copies can be obtained from orders@intechopen.com

Ulcerative Colitis - Etiology, Diagnosis, Diet, Special Populations, and the Role of Interventional Endoscopy
Edited by Partha Pal
p. cm.
Print ISBN 978-1-80355-294-1
Online ISBN 978-1-80355-295-8
eBook (PDF) ISBN 978-1-80355-296-5

For EU product safety concerns:
IN TECH d.o.o., Prolaz Marije Krucifikse Kozulić 3, 51000 Rijeka, Croatia,
info@intechopen.com or visit our website at intechopen.com.

Meet the editor

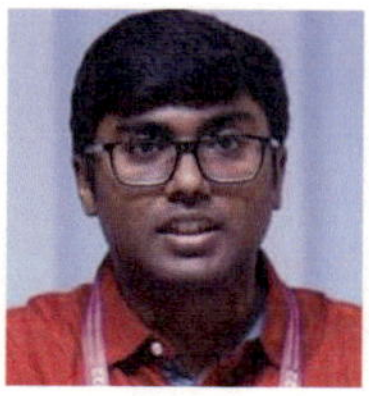

Dr. Partha Pal is a consultant gastroenterologist at the Asian Institute of Gastroenterology. He achieved high honors in his medical school and internal medicine training, receiving awards as the best student at the undergraduate and postgraduate levels. He has published over 60 peer-reviewed articles, mainly on interventional and clinical IBD, small bowel disease, interventional endoscopy, and pancreatic disease. He gained the National Young Scholar Award in 2017. Most recently he received the Endoscopic Training Award for the year 2021 from the American Society of GI endoscopy (ASGE) for his training work on interventional IBD and small bowel endoscopy.

Contents

Preface

Ulcerative colitis (UC), together with Crohn's disease (CD), is one of the major forms of inflammatory bowel disease (IBD). UC affects only the colon and rectum, while CD can affect any part of the bowel. Epidemiological trends suggest that in a region where IBD incidence is increasing, UC is the predominant subtype in the early years of increased industrialization, followed by a rise in the incidence of CD. This book covers various aspects of UC: etiology, clinical manifestation, histopathologic diagnosis, the role of anti-inflammatory dietary components such as fermented rice bran, special populations such as children and expectant mothers, the emerging role of interventional endoscopy in colitis-associated neoplasia, and the management of postoperative complications.

The etiology of UC is still unknown but it is multifactorial. In a genetically susceptible host, the combination of altered gut microbiome and environmental factors ultimately triggers the common pathway of dysregulated immune activation. First chapter, "Etiology of Ulcerative Colitis", discusses the well-known etiological factors that are unique to UC. The chapter "Platelets in Ulcerative Colitis: From Pathophysiology to Therapy" highlights the unique role of platelet activation in amplifying immune response in UC, and summarizes current evidence to support the role of anti-platelet therapy in UC.

Intestinal and extra-intestinal complications and manifestations are summarized with specific reference to pediatric patients in "Complications of Ulcerative Colitis in Children".

The two chapters "Histomorphological Diagnosis of Ulcerative Colitis and Associated Conditions" and "The Role of the Pathologist in Ulcerative Colitis" provide a concise illustrated review of all aspects of histopathology in UC. Histologic diagnosis of UC and histology in different stages of the disease are covered, together with histological scoring systems, histologic remission, differential diagnosis (from infective or Crohn's colitis), histopathological changes in special conditions (e.g., post-operative status, acute severe colitis), diagnosis of co-existent cytomegalovirus infection, and colitis-associated neoplasia.

Pediatric ulcerative colitis is a distinct subset of UC. Differences between pediatric and adult UC, natural history, diagnostic algorithms, and overall management, including acute severe UC and very early onset IBD (VEOIBD), are highlighted in the chapter "Pediatric Ulcerative Colitis".

Another special population in UC is pregnant women, a group that poses unique clinical challenges to the treating physician. Pre-conception planning (fertility, counseling, contraception, inducing remission), pregnancy care (obstetric, nutritional and drug therapy, management of flare and acute severe colitis, the role of endoscopy), and postpartum care (lactation, thromboprophylaxis, and contraception) are discussed in detail in the chapter "Ulcerative Colitis and Pregnancy".

As in Crohn's disease, anti-inflammatory diets are being explored in UC. "Dietary Fermented Rice Bran Is an Effective Modulator of Ulcerative Colitis in Experimental

Animals" highlights the potential role of anti-inflammatory dietary components in reducing gut permeability.

Finally, there is the emerging role of interventional endoscopy as a potential bridge between endoscopic and surgical therapy. The main indications in UC are endoscopic detection (using advanced endoscopic imaging) and resection of colitis-associated neoplasia, along with management of postoperative pouch complications. The chapter, "Role of Interventional IBD in Role of Interventional IBD in Management of Ulcerative Colitis(UC)-Associated Neoplasia and Post-Operative Pouch Complications in UC: A Systematic Review", is the first review of its kind and includes all currently available evidence for the role of interventional endoscopy in UC.

Ulcerative Colitis - Etiology, Diagnosis, Diet, Special Populations, and the Role of Interventional Endoscopy aims to act as a ready reference for the clinician treating ulcerative colitis. It provides indispensable updates on several relevant issues in the diagnosis and management of ulcerative colitis and has benefited from the collaboration of leading experts in various aspects of the disease. It aims to facilitate decision-making by gastroenterologists, IBD specialists, interventional endoscopists, dieticians, pathologists, surgeons, and pediatricians treating UC patients in their clinical practice.

Partha Pal
Asian Institute of Gastroenterology,
Department of Gastroenterology,
Hyderabad, India

Section 1

Ulcerative Colitis - Etiology

Chapter 1

Etiology of Ulcerative Colitis

Carmen-Monica Preda and Doina Istrătescu

Abstract

Ulcerative colitis (UC) is a chronic immune-mediated inflammatory disorder of the colon, related to a complex contribution of environmental and host factors that increase the susceptibility of individuals. Genetics, environmental factors, dysbiosis, and dysregulated immune system: all these components together are necessary to trigger IBD. The temporal sequence of events leading to UC is unknown. UC is not a classically transmitted genetic affliction. The risk of developing the disease is increased in first-degree relatives but there is no evidence that it is related to genetics or environmental factors exposure early in childhood. The environmental factors associated with ulcerative colitis development are diet, smoking, breastfeeding, use of antibiotics or NSAIDs, urban location, pollution exposure, appendectomy, and hypoxia. In normal intestinal homeostasis environment, both innate and adaptive immune systems are integrated with various mediators and immune cells to maintain tolerance to commensal organisms. In UC patients, the innate immune system is responsible for inducing inflammatory reactions, while the adaptive immune system is crucial in the evolution of chronic inflammatory events. With the shifting global burden of ulcerative colitis, more research is needed to better understand the illness's etiology in order to prevent and find potential novel therapeutic targets or predictors of disease burden in the future.

Keywords: ulcerative colitis, inflammatory bowel disease, etiology, genetics, environmental factors, immune response

1. Introduction

Ulcerative colitis (UC) is a chronic immune-mediated inflammatory disorder of the colon (IBD) that is hypothesized to be related to a complex contribution of environmental and host factors, that increase the susceptibility of individuals and events that damage the mucosal barrier, alter the gut microbiota's healthy balance, and inappropriately enhance gut immune responses, are all known to promote illness onset [1–3].

Despite knowing the pathophysiology of the disease, the exact etiology is not so clear, but it is likely to be multifactorial. Genetics, environmental factors, dysbiosis, and dysregulated immune system: all these components together are necessary to trigger IBD. The temporal sequence of events leading to UC is unknown up to now.

IntechOpen

2. Ulcerative colitis etiology

2.1 The role of genetics in UC

A number of genetic variables have been associated with ulcerative colitis. There are 163 susceptibility disease-associated loci associated with IBD. Thirty of them are associated with Crohn's disease (CD), 23 with ulcerative colitis and most of the remaining ones are common to both CD and UC, as well as other conditions: psoriasis, celiac disease [4, 5]. The unique genes associated with UC can be divided into genes that affect epithelial barrier (ECM1, HNF4A, CDH1, LAMB1, and GNA12), genes that are immune-mediated (IL8RA / IL8RB, IL2 / IL21, IFNG / IL26, IL7R, TNFRSF9, TNFRSF14, IRF5, LSP1, FCGR2A) and others (OTUD3 / PLA2G2E, PIM3, DAP, CAPN10, JAK2). The genes that overlap with Crohn's can also be divided into those that are immune-mediated: IL10, CARD9, MST1, ICOSLG, IL1R2, YDJC, PRDM1, TNFSF15, SMAD3, PTPN2, TNFRSF6B, HLA: DRB1*03 and others: ORMDL3, RTEL1/SLC2A4RG, PTGER4, KIF21B, NKX2-3, CREM, CDKAL1, STAT3, ZNF365, PSMG1, IL23R, IL12B, AK2, FUT2, and TYK2 [4, 6–9]. Further details are presented in **Tables 1–5** [4, 7, 9].

Recent studies have shown that the genes of the major histocompatibility complex are major genetic determinants of susceptibility to UC. The human leukocyte antigen (HLA) region on chromosome 6 is connected with the greatest genetic signals within UC-specific loci. Sixteen HLA allelic correlations for ulcerative colitis were revealed after further fine mapping genetic study, including HLA DRB1*01*03 for IBD colonic involvement [10, 11].

A unique yet rare missense mutation in the adenylate cyclase 7 gene (ADCY7) that doubles the risk of ulcerative colitis was discovered in a recent whole-genome sequencing study of over 2,000 ulcerative colitis patients. The ADCY7 gene has the strongest genetic connection with ulcerative colitis outside of the HLA area. ADCY7 is one of ten enzymes that convert ATP to cAMP. Additionally, numerous ulcerative colitis-specific genes are involved in epithelial barrier function regulation [12].

UC is not a classically transmitted genetic affliction. The risk of developing the disease is increased in first-degree relatives but there is no evidence that it is related to genetics or environmental factors exposure early in childhood or both conditions.

Gene	Locus	SNP	Protein name	Function
ECM1	1q21	rs3737240	Extracellular matrix protein 1	Involved in cell proliferation
HNF4A	20q13	rs6017342	Hepatocyte nuclear factor 4α	Regulates cellular differentiation along crypt-villus axis
CDH1	16q22	rs12597188	E-cadherin	Involved in epithelial adherens junction
LAMB1	7q31	rs886774	Laminin β1	Protein involved in cell adhesion and differentiation
GNA12	7p22	rs798502	guanine nucleotide-binding protein alpha 12	Protein is involved as modulators or transducers in various transmembrane signaling systems

Table 1.
Genes associated with UC that affect the epithelial barrier.

Gene	Locus	SNP	Protein name	Function
IL8RA / IL8RB	2q35	rs11676348	Interleukin 8 receptor alpha/ Interleukin 8 receptor beta	Activation of neutrophils
IL2 / IL21	4q27	rs17388568	Interleukin 2/ Interleukin 21	T-cell proliferation and other activities crucial to regulation of the immune response / Immunoregulatory activity. May promote the transition between innate and adaptive immunity
IFNG / IL26	12q14	rs7134599	Interferon gamma protein/ Interleukin 26	Cytokine is critical for innate and adaptive immunity/mucosal immunity, proinflammatory function
IL7R	5p13	rs3194051	Interleukin-7 receptor protein	Normal development of T cells
TNFRSF9	1p36	rs35675666	Tumor Necrosis Factor Receptor Superfamily Member 9	Co-stimulatory immune checkpoint molecule
TNFRSF14	1p36	rs10797432	Tumor necrosis factor receptor superfamily member 14	May mediate the signal transduction pathways that activate the immune response
IRF5	7q32	rs4728142	Interferon regulatory factor 5 protein	Transcription factor that plays a critical role in innate immunity
LSP1	11p15	rs907611	Lymphocyte-specific protein 1	Mediate neutrophil activation and chemotaxis
FCGR2A	1q23	rs1801274	Low-affinity immunoglobulin gamma Fc region receptor II-a protein	By binding to IgG it initiates cellular responses against pathogens and soluble antigens. Promotes phagocytosis of opsonized antigens.

Table 2.
Genes associated with UC—Immune-mediated.

Twin studies that compared the concordance rates of monozygotic and dizygotic twins backed up this conclusion. Monozygotic twins had a higher concordance (up to 17 percent in UC and up to 55 percent in CD) than dizygotic twins (6 percent in UC and 4 percent in CD), suggesting that the genetic trait is more important in Crohn's disease than ulcerative colitis. Furthermore, in both Crohn's disease and ulcerative colitis, genetic factors appear to differ across Western and Asian locations [13–18].

Another study reported a concordance rate among monozygotic twins of 67% for CD and 13–20% for UC; in one study, a lower rate of concordance for CD has been reported among monozygotic twins [19].

The overall lifetime risk (absolute risk) of developing IBD for first-degree relatives of a UC patient is 1.6% in non-Jews and 5.2% in Jews. Similarly, the risk (age-corrected) for offspring of a UC patient developing IBD is 11 and 2.9–7.4% in non-Jews and Jews, respectively. There is an increased risk (33–52%) in offspring with both affected parents [20].

However, there are many individuals that, when assessed by a polygenic risk score, do not present a genetic predisposition that accounts for all of the susceptibility loci. Despite the significance of genetic predisposition, no single genetic mutation can account for the rapid progression of UC. It is also unclear why some people with

Gene	Locus	SNP	Protein name	Function
OTUD3 / PLA2G2E	1p36	rs138347004	OTU Domain-Containing Protein 3 / Phosphatidylcholine 2-Acylhydrolase 2E	Protein turnover/role in inflammation and the immune response
PIM3	22q13	rs5771069	Serine/threonine-protein kinase pim-3	Prevent apoptosis, promote cell survival and protein translation
DAP	5p15	rs2930047	Death-associated protein 1	Negative regulator of autophagy. Involved in mediating interferon-gamma-induced cell death
CAPN10	2q37	rs4676410	Calcium-Activated Neutral Proteinase 10	Calcium-regulated non-lysosomal thiol-protease, which catalyzes limited proteolysis of substrates involved in cytoskeletal remodeling and signal transduction
JAK2	9p24	rs10758669	Tyrosine-Protein Kinase JAK2	Involved in cell growth, development, differentiation, or histone modifications. Mediates essential signaling events in both innate and adaptive immunity.

Table 3.
Other genes associated with UC.

Gene	Locus	SNP	Protein name	Function
IL10	1q32	rs3024505	Interleukin 10	Downregulates the expression of Th1 cytokines, MHC class II antigens, and co-stimulatory molecules on macrophages. It also enhances B cell survival, proliferation, and antibody production. IL-10 can block NF-κB activity and is involved in the regulation of the JAK-STAT signaling pathway
CARD9	9q34	rs10781499	Caspase recruitment domain-containing protein 9	Regulatory role in cell apoptosis
MST1	3p21	rs3197999	Macrophage-stimulating protein	Stimulates macrophages
ICOSLG	21q22	rs2838519	ICOS ligand	Co-stimulatory signal for T-cell proliferation and cytokine secretion; induces also B-cell proliferation and differentiation into plasma cells
IL1R2	2q11	rs2310173	Interleukin 1 receptor, type II	Binds interleukin alpha (IL1A), interleukin beta (IL1B), and interleukin 1 receptor, type I(IL1R1/IL1RA), and acts as a decoy receptor that inhibits the activity of its ligands

Gene	Locus	SNP	Protein name	Function
YDJC	22q11	rs181359	YdjC chitooligosaccharide deacetylase homolog	Predicted to enable deacetylase activity and magnesium ion binding activity. Predicted to be involved in carbohydrate metabolic process
PRDM1	6q21	rs6911490	PR domain zinc finger protein 1	Transcription factor regulating downstream cytokines. It is activated by TLRs and IRF-4 and is crucial in T cell, B cell, and myeloid lineage cell differentiations
TNFSF15	9q32	rs4246905	TNF superfamily member 15	It can activate both the NF-κB and MAPK signaling pathways and acts as an autocrine factor to induce apoptosis in endothelial cells
SMAD3	15q22	rs17293632	Mothers against decapentaplegic homolog 3	Up-regulation of genes and TGF-β-induced repression of target genes
PTPN2	18p11	rs1893217	Tyrosine-protein phosphatase non-receptor type 2	Involved in cell growth, differentiation, mitotic cycle, and oncogenic transformation
TNFRSF6B	20q13	rs6062504	Tumor necrosis factor receptor superfamily member 6B	Regulatory role in suppressing FasL- and LIGHT-mediated cell death and T cell activation
HLA:DRB1*03	6p21	rs9268853	Major histocompatibility complex, class II, DR beta 1	Displays foreign peptides to the immune system to trigger the body's immune response

Table 4.
Genes associated with IBD—Immune-mediated.

Gene	Locus	SNP	Protein name	Function
ORMDL3	17q12	rs2872507	ORMDL sphingolipid biosynthesis regulator 3	Negative regulation of B cell apoptotic process
RTEL1/ SLC2A4RG	20q13	rs2297441	Regulator of telomere elongation helicase 1/ SLC2A4 regulator	ATP-dependent DNA helicase is implicated in telomere-length regulation, DNA repair, and the maintenance of genomic stability. / transcription factor involved in SLC2A4 and HD gene transactivation
PTGER4	5p13	rs6451493	Prostaglandin E2 receptor 4	May play an important role in intestinal epithelial transport
KIF21B	1q32	rs7554511	Kinesin Family Member 21B	Plus-end-directed microtubule-dependent motor protein, which displays processive activity. Involved in delivery of gamma-aminobutyric acid (GABA(A)) receptor to the cell surface
NKX 2-3	10q24	rs6584283	Homeobox protein Nkx-2.3	Transcription factor

Gene	Locus	SNP	Protein name	Function
CREM	10p11	rs12261843	cAMP responsive element modulator	Bound to the -180 site of the IL-2 promoter to repress its transcription
CDKAL1	6p22	rs6908425	Cdk5 regulatory associated protein 1-like 1	Associated with adaptive immunity
STAT3	17q21	rs12942547	Signal transducer and activator of transcription 3	Essential for the differentiation of the TH17 helper T cells
ZNF365	10q21	rs10761659	Protein ZNF365	Contributes to genomic stability by preventing telomere dysfunction
PSMG1	21q22	rs9977672	Proteasome assembly chaperone 1	Enables proteasome binding
IL23R	1p31	rs11209026	Interleukin-23 receptor	Associates constitutively with Janus kinase 2 (JAK2) and also binds to transcription activator STAT3 in a ligand-dependent manner
IL12B	5q33	rs6871626	Subunit beta of interleukin 12	Sustain a sufficient number of memory/ effector Th1 cells to mediate long-term protection against an intracellular pathogen
AK2	1p35	rs804427	Adenylate Kinase 2	Catalyzes the reversible transfer of the terminal phosphate group between ATP and AMP
FUT2	19q13	rs516246	Galactoside 2-alpha-L-fucosyltransferase 2	regulates several processes such as cell-cell interaction including host-microbe interaction, cell surface expression, and cell proliferation
TYK2	19p13	rs11879191	Non-receptor tyrosine-protein kinase TYK2	Tyk2 is activated by IL-10, and its deficiency affects the ability to generate and respond to IL-10. Involved in the regulation of the JAK–STAT pathway

Table 5.
Other genes associated with IBD.

UC-associated risk variations remain healthy while others develop UC or perhaps several immune-mediated diseases [21, 22].

IBD susceptibility and progression cannot be explained solely by genetics. This indicates that abnormal adaptive immune responses and epithelial barrier dysfunction play a crucial role in disease development. Nongenetic factors, notably epigenetics, may have a role to play [23, 24]. A summary of the genetic factors that are associated with UC can be seen in **Table 6**.

Genetic predisposing factors for UC
HLA
ADCY7
67% of susceptibility loci are shared between UC and CD
Low disease hereditability in UC

Table 6.
Genetic predisposing factors for UC.

2.2 Environmental factors in UC

The rapid growth in the incidence of ulcerative colitis in newly industrialized nations implies that environmental factors have a role in disease initiation [25].

Ulcerative colitis comes initially in urban locations, with a quick rise in incidence followed by a slowing period. After that period, Crohn's disease grows in frequency, finally approaching that of UC. Industrialization is associated with a new urban lifestyle, pollution exposure, dietary changes, antibiotic access, improved cleanliness, and fewer infections, all of which are considered general contributory factors [26, 27]. Urbanization is no longer regarded as a risk factor, according to studies from both Western and developing jurisdictions [28–30].

2.2.1 Early life factors

Breast milk is often one of the first foods offered to babies. Breastfeeding has been shown in studies to help prevent the development of immune-mediated disorders by preserving the epithelial barrier, avoiding infections, and offering direct immunologic advantages [31–33]. A meta-analysis of 35 studies discovered a link between breastfeeding and the likelihood of developing ulcerative colitis later on [34].

Human milk oligosaccharides (HMOs), which are nondigestible molecules and free competitors to enteric pathogens, highly influence the composition of the infant gut microbiota. Formula-fed children's fecal microbiota is poorer in bifidobacteria and lactobacilli (only 40 to 60%), whereas breastfed children have a higher proportion of bacteria (90%). It demonstrates the important role of breast milk oligosaccharides in the establishment of the infant gut microbiota. HMOs are digested by gut bacteria and produce a variety of metabolites, including short-chain fatty acids (SCFA), which are well-known for their immunomodulatory characteristics. SCFA boosts numerous activities of the epithelial barrier after being absorbed by colonic epithelial cells. The mucus layer that covers epithelial cells is necessary for the epithelial barrier to remain intact. SCFA increases mucus production by upregulating mucin 2 expression, protects against inflammatory insults, and fortifies the tight junction barrier. They also modulate the inflammatory immune response by interacting with DC and T cells [35–38].

Hygiene hypothesis: evidence suggests an inverse relationship between the risk of UC and early childhood exposure to farm animals, pets, larger families, more siblings, and childbirth mode. As an internal environmental component, all of these early exposures are known to be major drivers for more diversified gut microbiota in early life. Although external variables are equally key determinants of health and disease, the positive relationship between the gut microbiota, host genetics, and immune system is an essential environmental factor in disease etiology [39–43].

Several studies have looked into whether antibiotic usage early in life predisposes to IBD in Western countries and have consistently shown this link [44]. According to a Canadian nested case-control study, 58 percent of juvenile IBD patients got antibiotics in their first year of life, compared to 39 percent of healthy controls. The number of antibiotic courses taken and the degree of the elevated risk of ulcerative colitis were also found to have a dose-response relationship [45]. Although the results of these studies are significant, other studies have failed to establish a relationship between the use of antibiotics and the risk of ulcerative colitis [46].

2.2.2 Adolescent influences

Quitting smoking has been linked to an increased risk of ulcerative colitis [47]. The pathophysiology of how smoking causes ulcerative colitis or protects a person from developing the condition is unknown. Active or passive smoking produces milder forms of the disease in the case of UC, requiring fewer surgeries throughout its development and less need for immunosuppressive drugs. It is unclear whether the rise in ulcerative colitis is related to smoking cessation patterns. Indian research shows that there is no link between quitting smoking and the development of ulcerative colitis. As for the association between active smoking and the incidence of Crohn's disease, there is also no evidence in their studies [30, 48].

Studies proposed the divergent effect of appendectomy on UC suggesting inflammation of appendix might have protective interplay with the disease [49, 50].

The dietary habits of adolescents are characterized by excessive consumption of meat and fat and an insufficient intake of fiber, fruits, and vegetables. There is also a tendency to frequently consume processed food and high sugary or soft drinks that increase the risk of developing IBD [51]. This subject will be further discussed in the Diet chapter.

Stress and distress can cause depression and anxiety. Psychological comorbidity is three times higher in those with IBD than in the general population. More than a quarter of people with IBD will have depression at some point in their lives, and more than a third will experience anxiety. Not only does having this chronic disease cause an increase in anxiety and depression but it is also possible that having these psychiatric disorders makes you more likely to develop IBD. It is unclear how much depression and IBD have in common in terms of gene alterations, epigenetic changes, or immunological responses. When they coexist, it has a detrimental influence on health-related quality of life (HRQOL), regardless of which arrives first: impaired mental health or IBD [52–54].

2.2.3 Other factors

NSAIDs are among the most commonly used drugs, and their link to ulcers in the stomach or duodenum is well known. They have, however, been associated with the development of IBD. Several theories have been proposed as possible mechanisms for the link between NSAIDs and IBD. A prospective cohort study assessed the link between aspirin and nonsteroidal anti-inflammatory drug (NSAID) use and the occurrence of Crohn's disease and ulcerative colitis. A higher risk of both conditions was observed with the highest frequency of NSAID use [55].

In urban areas, air pollution has been related to a variety of health problems. In mice, acute exposure to high levels of airborne particulate matter increases gut permeability and heightens the innate immune response in the small intestine, while chronic exposure results in increased expression of pro-inflammatory cytokines and changes in colon microbiota composition and function. Long-term exposure also aggravated colitis in an Il10/mouse model [56].

Particulate matter exposure has given inconsistent results in epidemiological studies evaluating the link between air pollution and ulcerative colitis, showing that when there is a link, other components of air pollution may play a role in disease development. People who lived in locations with greater SO2 concentrations were more likely to develop ulcerative colitis than people who lived in areas with lower SO2 concentrations [57]. In a European nested case-control study, airborne particulate

Environmental factors in UC
Smoking
Appendectomy
Breastfeeding
Antibiotic usage in childhood
NSAIDs
Air pollution
Hypoxia

Table 7.
Summary of environmental factors in UC.

matter interaction was found to be inversely related to the incidence of IBD, but not Crohn's disease or ulcerative colitis. In contrast, living near a high-traffic area was linked to a higher risk of disease, and other air pollutants such as nitrous oxides had a trend toward positive relationships with IBD [58].

Hypoxia has been shown to cause inflammatory responses in immune and endothelial cells, with a buildup of inflammatory cells in different organs and increased cytokines in experimental animal models after short-term exposure to low oxygen levels. Levels of circulating IL-6, IL-1ra, and C-reactive protein are elevated in human studies in response to hypobaric hypoxic settings such as high altitudes, and the systemic elevations in these inflammatory markers could reflect local inflammation in the intestine [59, 60].

Hypoxia-inducible factor (HIF), a transcription factor that is dormant when oxygen is available but activated in hypoxic situations, is required for cellular responses to hypoxia. Patients with ulcerative colitis or Crohn's disease have increased expression of HIF-1. Patients with IBD also have increased colonic mRNA expression of glycolytic enzymes, which is triggered by hypoxia through the transcription factor HIF-1 [59, 61].

Based on the hypothesis that hypoxia leads to intestinal inflammation, a small pilot proof-of-concept randomized trial that included 18 patients demonstrated hyperbaric oxygen therapy to be beneficial in moderate-to-severe ulcerative colitis (**Table 7**) [62].

2.3 Diet

Multiple epidemiological researchers have concluded a link between nutrition and ulcerative colitis. In recent decades, significant changes in food intake have been related to an increase in the incidence of UC. Consumption of soft drinks and sucrose was linked to an increased chance of acquiring the condition. On the other hand, the consumption of fruits and vegetables was related to a decrease in UC development [63–68].

There is a significant association between red meat intake and ulcerative colitis risk [69]. Furthermore, whereas dietary n-3 polyunsaturated fatty acids (PUFAs) were linked to a lower risk of UC (odds ratio: 0.56) [70], dietary arachidonic acid (an n-6 PUFA) assessed in adipose tissue was linked to a higher risk of UC (relative risk: 4.16) [71].

Although there is no evidence of the mechanisms involved in the diet role in IBD development, there are several plausible explanations such as the effects on composition of gut microbiota, the microbial metabolites produced, and alterations in mucosal barrier and immunity [72].

Diet plays a major role in the composition of gut microbiota. Several studies demonstrated that a change in the gut microbiome induced by diet can result in a disease-inducing entity that could either initiate or perpetuate inflammation in patients with IBD. Differences in food patterns between African and European children were related to increased Bacteroidetes and decreased Firmicutes and Enterobacteriaceae [73, 74].

A high fat/high sugar diet can result in intestinal mucosal dysbiosis characterized by an overgrowth of pro-inflammatory proteobacteria and a decrease in protective bacteria. Dietary factors have significant effects on microbial composition and can also affect the metabolic functions of gut microbiota. In both small and large intestines, commensal bacterial fermentation of indigestible food fibers produces short chain fatty acids (SCFA). SCFA changes gene expression, cellular differentiation, chemotaxis, proliferation, and apoptosis in epithelial and/or immunological cells [75]. Some UC patients have a lower amount of SCFA-producing bacteria such as Faecalibacterium prausnitzii, which is inversely connected to disease activity. Furthermore, experimental investigations have linked a western diet high in sugar and fat and low in dietary fiber to lower SCFAs and greater colitis susceptibility [76–78].

There have been demonstrated links between dietary PUFA content and inflammatory processes in IBD. Dietary n-3 polyunsaturated fatty acid (PUFA) intake has been linked to a lower risk of ulcerative colitis, while dietary n-6 PUFA intake has been linked to a higher risk of ulcerative colitis [71, 79, 80]. Dietary n-3 PUFAs reduced the clinical severity of spontaneous and NSAID-induced colitis in rats. Furthermore, TNF generated by splenic CD4+ T cells was inhibited. These findings are consistent with previous reports establishing the preventive impact of n-3 PUFAs on experimental colitis [81], as TNF plays a key role in IBD development.

Dietary variables may have a direct impact on the cells of the host. Some studies have demonstrated that luminal iron may affect the function of intestinal epithelial cells and T cells and also triggers the apoptosis of epithelial cell stress [82]. Zinc deficiency can also decrease the barrier integrity and increase the permeability in IBD patients and vitamin D has a role in reducing inflammation in experimental and human IBD [83, 84].

Several food additives, such as emulsifying agents, maltodextrin, and thickeners including carrageenan, carboxymethyl cellulose, and xanthan gum, have been shown to disrupt intestinal homeostasis [85]. Carrageenan is a type of sulfated polysaccharide derived from seaweed. The US Food and Drug Administration has approved it as "generally regarded as safe," and it is utilized in the food industry for its gelling, thickening, and stabilizing characteristics. Reduced protein and peptide bioaccessibility, disturbance of normal epithelial function, and intestinal inflammation have all been associated with carrageenan [86]. Within one day, carboxymethyl cellulose and polysorbate80 were found to shift the gut microbiota into a pro-inflammatory state by raising bioactive flagellin levels. Changes in gene expression and the development of colitis have been linked to the pro-inflammatory microbiota [87, 88].

Other studies have found that complete dietary guidance, low FODMAP, or IgG-guided exclusion diets are useful in reducing disease activity in UC patients [89–91]. Although these findings are encouraging, one of the significant limitations of these studies is that they did not disclose their findings separately for patients with active disease and those in remission, making it difficult to make meaningful judgments (**Table 8**).

Increased risk	Decreased risk
Soft drinks	Fruits
Sucrose	Vegetables
Red meat	n-3 PUFAs
n-6 PUFAs	Normal levels of vitamin D
Food additives	Low FODMAP
Zinc deficiency	Diet guidance
Luminal iron exposure	IgG-guided exclusion diet

Table 8.
Dietary factors associated with an increased/decreased risk of developing UC.

2.4 Microbiome

Early gut microbial colonization is integral to the development of the immune system and intestinal homeostasis, providing a synergistic relationship between defensive and tolerant mechanisms [92]. Different studies from the literature have demonstrated that patients with ulcerative colitis have disturbances in the composition of their gut microbiota, coined "microbial dysbiosis," with a reduction in bacterial diversity with lower proportions of Firmicutes (phylum) and Bacteroides (genus) and higher proportions of Enterobacteriaceae (family) [73, 93–95]. Short-chain fatty acid (SCFA)-producing Ruminococcaceae and Lachnospiraceae have been shown to be depleted, whereas pro-inflammatory microorganisms such as Enterobacteriaceae, especially Escherichia coli and Fusobacteriaceae have grown in number [96, 97].

It is unclear if dysbiosis is a result of or a cause of gut inflammation in ulcerative colitis. In ulcerative colitis, the virome and mycobiome are similarly less varied in this regard [98–101]. There are four controlled positive faecal microbial transplantation clinical studies that confirm the therapeutic effect for ulcerative colitis patients [102–105]. Microbial diversity restoration, particularly the bacterial species responsible for SCFA generation in donor stool, has been indicated as a key factor [102, 106].

In ulcerative colitis, one of the main impacts of dysbiosis is likely to be a decline in the epithelium health or a state of epithelial malfunction, which increases inherent sensitivity to disease. Faecal diversion away from the rectum worsens inflammation, resulting in "diversion colitis" in ulcerative colitis; on the other hand, faecal diversion decreases inflammation in Crohn's disease [107].

The microbiome is the most unstable during childhood, and disturbances to the microbiota in the earliest years of life may alter gut immunity and, therefore,

Decreased diversity of UC gut microbiome, virome, and mycobiome over time
dysbiosis: either a result or a cause of gut inflammation in ulcerative colitis
Imbalance: ↓ protective microbes (Firmicutes and Bacteroides) / ↑ inflammatory microbes (Enterobacteriaceae and Fusobacteriaceae)
Dysbiosis in the earliest years of life → alteration of gut immunity → ↑ susceptibility to IBD

Table 9.
Overview of microbiota changes in UC.

susceptibility to IBD [108]. Before, during, and after a 5-day treatment with oral ciprofloxacin, the variety, richness, and evenness of the faecal microbiota in healthy humans were reduced [109]. Because antibiotics are widely used in both developing and developed countries and are progressively used in poor countries, it is plausible to believe that antibiotic use is a fundamental predisposing factor in IBD etiology. Antibiotic misuse and abuse, as well as their usage in cattle, could aggravate the problem (**Table 9**).

2.5 Epithelial barrier alteration

An increased population of effector T cells and increased production of proinflammatory cytokines (such as TNF- α, IL-6, and IFN- γ) are thought to be the cause of ulcerative colitis. The balance between proinflammatory and immunosuppressive forces can determine the progression of inflammation that is characteristic of IBD. Disruption of intestinal homeostasis can be determined by an epithelial barrier deficiency. This deficiency has multiple causes: a primary dysbiosis of the intestinal microbiota, a defect in the mucus layer, a primary defect of the epithelium, or an inflamed state of the lamina propria [110].

An epithelial barrier deficiency is seen early in the etiology of UC. For example, in individuals with active UC, the thickness of the mucin-containing mucosal layer of the colon has been demonstrated to be reduced, primarily due to decreased mucin 2 synthesis. In addition, in the early stages of UC, although the epithelium looks normal endoscopically, apoptotic foci can already be observed. This weakened barrier function might be caused by a fundamental genetic deficiency or environmental influences such as changes in the microbiota [111].

Susceptibility polymorphisms in genes producing junctional proteins such as E-cadherin, guanine nucleotide-binding protein alpha 12, and Zonula occludens-1 have been found in genome-wide association studies (GWAS), suggesting that epithelial barrier abnormalities may be a major cause for UC. Furthermore, alterations in the expression of junctional proteins such as E-cadherin, b-catenin, and claudins have been detected in intestinal biopsies from patients with IBD, indicating that barrier disruption plays a role in IBD etiology [112, 113].

2.6 Immune response in UC

Because the human immune system is responsible for recognizing, responding to, and adapting to a wide range of self and foreign molecules, its integrity is vital for maintaining and recovering health. In the gastrointestinal system, there are two complicated mucosal immune processes that check the luminal contents on a regular basis, recognize microbial or dietary antigens, and activate immune pathways. During the active phase of gut diseases, such as UC, both innate and adaptive immune systems are integrated with various mediators and immune cells to maintain tolerance, manage low-grade inflammation, and upregulate [114].

Antigen-presenting cells (APCs) include dendritic cells, B cells, and macrophages, which are important in both innate and adaptive immunity and immune homeostasis because they can secrete cytokines and activate innate immunity while also presenting antigens to adaptive immune cells, thus linking adaptive and innate immunity pathways [115].

2.6.1 Innate immune response

Innate immunity consists of defense-related elements that are programmed or automatic, such as the mucosal barrier, epithelial cell tight junctions, and gut permeability control, as well as the secretion of antimicrobial enzymes like defensins and lysozyme to protect the lamina propria from microbial raids. The innate immune system is composed of macrophages, monocytes, neutrophils, and other granulocytes, as well as natural killer cells (NKs), dendritic cells, mast cells, and innate lymphoid cells (ILCs). Non-immune cells involved in the innate immunity system include intestinal epithelial cells (IECs), endothelial cells, transforming growth factor-releasing stromal cells, and mesenchymal cells [116].

Several types of innate immune cells have been implicated in the development of IBD. Neutrophils contribute to the persistence of intestinal inflammation by impairing epithelial barrier function and releasing numerous inflammatory mediators. To maintain homeostasis, dendritic cells (DCs) regulate crosstalk between innate and adaptive immunity. In IBD, however, inappropriate conditioning of DCs has been observed throughout both active and passive disease states as a result of decreased mucosal expression of TGF-b and TSLP, as well as downregulation of the retinoic acid signaling pathway [115].

Macrophages and DCs, as well as epithelial cells and myofibroblasts, maintain gut immunological homeostasis by continuously recognizing microbial antigens. Mucosal DCs and macrophages from IBD patients have higher levels of TLR2, TLR4, CD40, and the chemokine receptor CCR7, all of which contribute to and promote inflammation by stimulating the release of pro-inflammatory cytokines like TNF, IL-1b, IL-6, and IL-18 [114–116].

2.6.2 Adaptive immune response

Adaptive immunity is characterized by unique immunological responses triggered by antigen-specific activation of B cells or T cells. This immune system includes antibody-secreting B cells, cytotoxic T cells, effector T cells, regulatory T cells (Tregs), and T helper lymphocytes that are all engaged in this process. Peyer's patches of the small intestine, lymphoid follicles of the colon, and mesenteric lymph nodes are the places where adaptive immune cells differentiate. The human immune system's basic function is determined by its interaction with the human microbiome [9].

Several types of innate immune cells have been implicated in the development of IBD. Neutrophils contribute to intestinal inflammation by impairing epithelial barrier function and secreting a variety of inflammatory mediators. To maintain homeostasis, dendritic cells (DCs) regulate crosstalk between innate and adaptive immunity. Intestinal epithelial cells that generate retinoic acid, thymic stromal lymphopoietin (TSLP), and transforming growth factor (TGF)- β impact DCs, increasing the formation of IL-10-producing DCs and thus anti-inflammatory responses and tolerance. In both active and inactive IBD disease stages, decreased mucosal expression of TGF- β and TSLP, as well as downregulation of the retinoic acid signaling pathway, leads to improper conditioning of DCs. [117].

A complex inflammatory process involving innate and adaptive immune cells entering the lamina propria occurs during the active phase of UC. Neutrophils, the short-lived "first responder" cells, are recruited in large numbers with the histology of "crypt abscesses," and they migrate over the epithelium before dying in the crypts. [118].

The survival of neutrophils is aided by the inflammatory environment (potentially via HIF-1 and hypoxia). As a result of this prolonged survivability, its inflammatory impact and tissue damage are intensified (via many means, including the release of serine and matrix metalloproteases, reactive oxygen species, and pro-inflammatory cytokines). Uncontrolled pro-inflammatory cell death (necrosis, necroptosis, and NETosis) occurs in a large proportion of neutrophils, amplifying and potentiating the pro-inflammatory milieu. High quantities of s100a8/9 proteins (or calprotectin) produced in blood and stool, as well as a strong serological response to self peri-nuclear anti p-neutrophil cytoplasmic antibodies (pANCA), are both likely indirect indications of uncontrolled neutrophil cell death, corroborate this mechanism in UC. Extracellular traps (NETs) on neutrophils can operate as a net for immunogenic chemicals that keep the inflammatory response going. All of these changes support the rational paradigm that, following the onset of the disease, a wave of innate inflammatory neutrophils and monocytes (with their pro-inflammatory cytokine repertoire, such as IL-1 family, IL-6, and TNF- α) creates an inflammatory environment (nutritional, metabolic, and cytokine) that promotes a pathologic adaptive (likely T-cell) immune response [119–121].

All of these parameters will influence the host's ability to resolve inflammation, restore homeostasis, and heal the UC mucosa, as well as newly incoming inflammatory monocytes, monocyte-macrophage activity, survival, and phenotype [122].

Because of UC's significant genetic connections to HLA (mainly class II), defective antigen(s) drive the aberrant T-cell response, which subsequently shapes the pathologic cytokine milieu, and is considered to be a key causal component. The complete mechanism of how HLA affects commensal and/or self-antigen presentation to T cells, and then a downstream pathogenic T-cell response, is yet unknown and difficult to understand. Approaches to studying, screening, and defining T-cell epitopes have vastly improved, and further development is expected [123].

Naïve CD4+ T-cells activated by antigen-specific signals from APCs, influenced by the cytokine milieu, differentiate into effector T-helper cells; T-helper 1 (Th1), T-helper 2 (Th2), T-helper 17 (Th17) cells, T-helper 9 (Th9), or regulatory T-cells (Tregs). Previously, it was thought that the differentiation of naive CD4+ T-cells into effector T-cell lineages was an irreversible process; however, specific cytokine circumstances and stimuli may cause plasticity between T-cell subsets [124]. Treg and Th17 plasticity are most likely triggered by dynamic changes in the inflammatory environment. As a result, pro-inflammatory stimuli may stimulate the conversion of immune-suppressive regulatory T cells into pro-inflammatory Th17 cells, while inflammation resolution may induce or even necessitate the switch from Th17 to Treg [125].

UC is traditionally associated with a Th2 response characterized by high levels of IL-4, IL-5, and IL-13, whereas CD is characterized by a Th1/Th17 response. Previous research has linked UC to a nonclassical Th2 response, with CD1d-restricted natural killer T-cells releasing IL-13. This region has been overwhelmed by subsequent developments. The discovery of IL-23 as a critical driver of Th17 responses, genetic connections with IL-23 and associated genes and the presence of Th17 (and Th9) cells in UC are only a few examples. IL-9 is produced from Th9 cells, a new subtype of Th cells. Th9 cells develop from naïve T cells under the induction of transforming growth factor (TGF)-β and IL-4. IL-9 is thought to disrupt gut barrier function by inhibiting intestinal epithelial cell proliferation and suppressing the expression of many tight-junction proteins such as claudin and occludin. Furthermore, greater IL-9 levels in UC patients with

Pathogenic adaptive (presumably T-cell driven) responses: triggered by innate immune responses (neutrophils/macrophages)
HLA allelic connections may influence antigen presentation
Complex UC immunity: • a nonclassical Th2 response • Th9 response • Th17 response • interleukin (IL)-23 inflammatory pathway

Table 10.
Overview of the immune responses in UC.

severe disease compared to patients with moderate disease and control patients may represent disease activity, as seen by the higher IL-9 levels reported in UC patients with severe disease compared to patients with mild disease and control patients [126–128].

Multiple pathways occur in the recruitment of mesenchymal cells and the formation of activated myofibroblasts, the major functional unit responsible for excessive extracellular matrix (ECM) deposition, during intestinal injury and repair. Multiple matrix metalloproteinases (MMPs) are significantly expressed in IBD tissues, with interstitial collagenase (MMP1) and MMP2 mediating collagen fiber breakdown, whereas fistula formation in Crohn's disease has been linked to elevated expression of MMP3 and MMP9. A balance between MMPs and tissue inhibitors of metalloproteinase occurs, resulting in excessive deposition of certain ECM components. All of these anomalies are most likely the result of inflammation-derived soluble mediators that regulate ECM deposition.

Primary human intestinal epithelial cells (IECs) from normal mucosa may process and deliver antigens to primed peripheral blood CD8+ T lymphocytes that act as nonspecific suppressor cells. IBD-associated IECs have a reduced ability to induce CD8+ T suppressor cells, implying a deficiency in mucosal immunoregulation that predisposes to IBD [129].

Despite the fact that CD4 T cells are thought to have a larger role in IBD pathogenesis, CD8 T cell transcriptomic patterns have been identified to determine whether UC follows a more aggressive course. The recent discovery of innate lymphoid cells (ILCs) as a further mediator of IL-23-driven inflammatory response in the colon is a further new dimension in UC [130–132].

While the innate immune system is responsible for inducing inflammatory reactions, the adaptive immune system is crucial in the evolution of chronic inflammatory events in UC (**Table 10**).

2.7 New advances in the etiology

Recent studies suggest that mitochondria have a major role in inflammation. Mitochondrial dysfunction has long been linked to UC, but recent paper released in the last three years has re-emphasized this theory. Earlier colonic microarray investigations in UC revealed such dysregulation of genes that affect mitochondrial activity [133–135].

When mitochondrial homeostasis is disrupted, energy generation is impaired, mitochondrial oxidative stress rises, and mitochondrial products (mitochondrial DNA) are released as pro-inflammatory DAMPs. All of these factors play a role in core UC themes such as epithelial failure, the pro-inflammatory mucosal environment, and direct inflammatory triggers. As a result of this convergence of facts, novel techniques for targeting pro-inflammatory mitochondria have emerged, such as mitochondrial antioxidant therapy in active UC [136, 137].

Inflammation causes tissue damage and different forms of cell death (apoptosis, necrosis, necroptosis, and pyroptosis), as well as the release of several cytosolic and nuclear products with intrinsic proinflammatory characteristics, as seen in IBD. DAMPs are the term used to describe those items. Proteins and peptides (High mobility group box 1 protein [HMGB1], defensins, heat-shock proteins, S100 proteins, IL1 and IL33, and so on), lipoproteins and fatty acids (such as serum amyloid A and oxidized low-density lipoproteins), ECM degradation products (for example, hyaluronan fragments), and nucleic acids are among the many different types of DAMPs. Through a DAMP-mediated mechanism, any agent, medicine, or virus that damages the epithelium can cause IBD flare-ups and clinical illness recurrence [138].

Exogenous, microbial, stress, and endogenous danger signals trigger inflammasomes, which activate caspase 1 and produce IL1 and IL18. Inflammasomes are members of the NLR or pyrin family, with members of the NOD-like receptor family, such as NLRP1a/b, NLRP3, NLRC4, and AIM2, regulating immunological responses, metabolism, and disease pathogenesis being the best known. The inflammasome's function in regulating interaction between the mucosal immune system and the microbiota makes it particularly appealing and biologically relevant to IBD immunopathogenesis. Inflammasome activity appears to be higher in CD based on circumstantial data, but there is no information available for UC [139].

MicroRNAs (miRNAs) are single-stranded noncoding RNAs with key regulatory activities on gene expression, primarily via suppressing (silencing) genes via degradation of target RNAs or translation inhibition. Long noncoding RNAs and circular RNAs are two more forms of noncoding RNAs that have been discovered. These noncoding RNAs also have important regulatory activities, and how these functions may be involved in IBD pathogenesis is becoming a hot topic. Excessive immunological reactivity and inflammation, both of which are linked to IBD, could be caused by dysregulation or insufficient miRNA-mediated repression [140].

Single-cell profiling of the inflamed UC mucosa allows for a thorough examination and census of the cell populations. New research has discovered new and unusual cell kinds, as well as cell-type-specific expression and deep cell–cell interactions and cell lineage linkages. Mucosal compartments that have gotten less attention in the past, such as the colonic mesenchyme, are now being identified as major mediators of inflammation, but all of this needs to be confirmed in the future (**Table 11**) [141–143].

Disruption of mitochondrial homeostasis → alteration of energy production →↑ oxidative stress →release of pro-inflammatory damage-associated molecular patterns.
Novel techniques in active UC: targeting pro-inflammatory mitochondria, (i.e. mitochondrial antioxidant therapy)
Major mediators of inflammation: colonic mesenchyme

Table 11.
New advances in UC.

3. Conclusion

Despite recent advances in our understanding of the role of environmental exposures, genetics, dysbiosis, and dysregulated immunity in disease development, the temporal sequence of events leading to IBD remains unknown. They are all important in triggering IBD/UC because none of the factors alone can cause IBD/UC. Immune system is the effector arm for inflammatory response. With the shifting global burden of ulcerative colitis, more research is needed to better understand the illness's etiology in order to prevent and find potential novel therapeutic targets or predictors of disease burden in the future.

Acknowledgements

I would like to express my deep and sincere gratitude to my mentors MD, Ph.D. in gastroenterology and internal medicine, Chief of Gastroenterology and Hepatology Department, Fundeni Clinical Institute, Mircea Mihai Diculescu, and MD, Ph.D. in gastroenterology and internal medicine, Ioan-Alexandru Oproiu for their support and helpful feedback throughout the years.

Conflict of interest

The authors declare no conflict of interest.

Author details

Carmen-Monica Preda* and Doina Istrătescu
Department of Gastroenterology and Hepatology, Fundeni Clinical Institute, "Carol Davila" University of Medicine and Pharmacy, Bucharest, Romania

*Address all correspondence to: carmenmonica.preda@gmail.com

References

[1] Abraham BP, Kane S. Fecal markers: Calprotectin and lactoferrin. Gastroenterology Clinical North America. 2012;**41**:483-495

[2] Ng SC, Bernstein CN, Vatn MH, et al. Geographical variability and environmental risk factors in inflammatory bowel disease. Gut. 2013;**62**:630-649

[3] Porter RJ, Kalla R, Ho GT. Ulcerative colitis: Recent advances in the understanding of disease pathogenesis. F1000Res. 2020;**9**:294

[4] Jostins L, Ripke S, Weersma RK, et al. Host-microbe interactions have shaped the genetic architecture of inflammatory bowel disease. Nature. 2012;**491**(7422):119-124

[5] Dobre M, Mănuc TE, Milanesi E, et al. Mucosal CCR1 gene expression as a marker of molecular activity in Crohn's disease: Preliminary data. Romanian Journal of Morphology and Embryology. 2017;**58**(4):1263-1268

[6] de Lange KM, Barrett JC. Understanding inflammatory bowel disease via immunogenetics. Journal of Autoimmunity. 2015;**64**:91-100

[7] Kaur A, Goggolidou P. Ulcerative colitis: Understanding its cellular pathology could provide insights into novel therapies. Journal of Inflammation. 2020;**17**:15

[8] Cho JH. The genetics and immunopathogenesis of inflammatory bowel disease. Nature Reviews. Immunology. 2008;**8**(6):458-466

[9] Anderson CA, Boucher G, Lees CW, et al. Meta-analysis identifies 29 additional ulcerative colitis risk loci, increasing the number of confirmed associations to 47. Nature Genetics. 2011;**43**(3):246-252

[10] Goyette P, Boucher G, Mallon D, et al. High-density mapping of the MHC identifies a shared role for HLA-DRB1*01:03 in inflammatory bowel diseases and heterozygous advantage in ulcerative colitis. Nature Genetics. 2015;**47**(2):172-179

[11] Ţieranu CG, Dobre M, Mănuc TE, et al. Gene expression profile of endoscopically active and inactive ulcerative colitis: Preliminary data. Romanian Journal of Morphology and Embryology. 2017;**58**(4):1301-1307

[12] Luo Y, de Lange KM, Jostins L, et al. Exploring the genetic architecture of inflammatory bowel disease by whole-genome sequencing identifies association at ADCY7. Nature Genetics. 2017;**49**(2):186-192

[13] Spehlmann ME, Begun AZ, Saroglou E, et al. Risk factors in German twins with inflammatory bowel disease: Results of a questionnaire-based survey. Journal of Crohn's & Colitis. 2012;**6**(1):29-42

[14] Halfvarson J, Bodin L, Tysk C, Lindberg E, Järnerot G. Inflammatory bowel disease in a Swedish twin cohort: A long-term follow-up of concordance and clinical characteristics. Gastroenterology. 2003;**124**(7):1767-1773

[15] Ng SC, Woodrow S, Patel N, Subhani J, Harbord M. Role of genetic and environmental factors in British twins with inflammatory bowel disease. Inflammatory Bowel Diseases. 2012;**18**(4):725-736

[16] van Dongen J, Slagboom PE, Draisma HH, Martin NG, Boomsma DI. The continuing value of twin studies in the omics era. Nature Reviews. Genetics. 2012;**13**(9):640-653

[17] Yoshitake S, Kimura A, Okada M, Yao T, Sasazuki T. HLA class II alleles in Japanese patients with inflammatory bowel disease. Tissue Antigens. 1999;**53**(4 Pt 1):350-358

[18] Inoue N, Tamura K, Kinouchi Y, et al. Lack of common NOD2 variants in Japanese patients with Crohn'sdisease. Gastroenterology. 2002;**123**(1):86-91

[19] Yang H, McElree C, Roth MP, Shanahan F, Targan SR, Rotter JI. Familial empirical risks for inflammatory bowel disease: Differences between Jews and non-Jews. Gut. 1993;**34**(4):517-524

[20] Hedin C. Molecular genetics of inflammatory bowel disease. D'Amato M, Rioux JD, editors. Springer; 2013

[21] Manuc M, Ionescu EM, Milanesi E, et al. Molecular signature of persistent histological inflammation in ulcerative colitis with mucosal healing. Journal of Gastrointestinal and Liver Diseases. 2020;**29**(2):159-166

[22] Lee HS, Cleynen I. Molecular profiling of inflammatory bowel disease: Is it ready for use in clinical decision-making? Cell. 2019;**8**(6):535

[23] Ventham NT, Kennedy NA, Nimmo ER, Satsangi J. Beyond gene discovery in inflammatory bowel disease: The emerging role of epigenetics. Gastroenterology. 2013;**145**(2):293-308

[24] Kalla R, Ventham NT, Kennedy NA. MicroRNAs: New players in inflammatory bowel disease. Gut. 2015;**64**(6):1008

[25] Ng SC, Shi HY, Hamidi N, et al. Worldwide incidence and prevalence of inflammatory bowel disease in the 21st century: A systematic review of population-based studies. Lancet. 2017;**390**(10114):2769-2778

[26] Kirsner JB. Historical aspects of inflammatory bowel disease. Journal of Clinical Gastroenterology. 1998;**10**(3):286-297

[27] Kaplan GG, Ng SC. Understanding and preventing the global increase of inflammatory bowel disease. Gastroenterology. 2017;**152**(2):313-321

[28] Wang YF, Ou-Yang Q, Xia B, et al. Multicenter case-control study of the risk factors for ulcerative colitis in China. World Journal of Gastroenterology. 2013;**19**(11):1827-1833

[29] Benchimol EI, Kaplan GG, Otley AR, et al. Rural and urban residence during early life is associated with risk of inflammatory bowel disease: A population-based inception and birth cohort study. The American Journal of Gastroenterology. 2017;**112**(9):1412-1422

[30] Amarapurkar AD, Amarapurkar DN, Rathi P, et al. Risk factors for inflammatory bowel disease: A prospective multi-center study. Indian Journal of Gastroenterology. 2018;**37**(3):189-195

[31] Parigi SM, Eldh M, Larssen P, Gabrielsson S, Villablanca EJ. Breast milk and solid food shaping intestinal immunity. Frontiers in Immunology. 2015;**6**:415

[32] Renz H, Brandtzaeg P, Hornef M. The impact of perinatal immune development on mucosal homeostasis and chronic inflammation. Natural Review in Immunology. 2011;**12**:9

[33] Rogier EW, Frantz AL, Bruno ME, et al. Lessons from mother: Long-term impact of antibodies in breast milk on the gut microbiota and intestinal immune system of breastfed offspring. Gut Microbes. 2014;**5**(5):663-668

[34] Xu L, Lochhead P, Ko Y, Claggett B, Leong RW, Ananthakrishnan AN. Systematic review with meta-analysis: Breastfeeding and the risk of Crohn's disease and ulcerative colitis. Aliment Pharmacology Therapy. 2017;**46**(9):780-789

[35] Hegar B, Wibowo Y, Basrowi RW, et al. The role of two human milk oligosaccharides, 2'-Fucosyllactose and Lacto-N-Neotetraose, in infant nutrition. Pediatric Gastroenterology Hepatology Nutrition. 2019;**22**:330-340

[36] Harmsen HJ, Wildeboer-Veloo AC, Raangs GC, et al. Analysis of intestinal flora development in breast-fed and formula-fed infants by using molecular identification and detection methods. Journal of Pediatric Gastroenterology and Nutrition. 2000;**30**:61-67

[37] Boudry G, Charton E, Le Huerou-Luron I, et al. The relationship between breast milk components and the infant gut microbiota. Frontiers in Nutrition. 2021;**8**:629740

[38] Zuurveld M, van Witzenburg NP, Garssen J, et al. Immunomodulation by human milk oligosaccharides: The potential role in prevention of allergic diseases. Frontiers in Immunology. 2020;**11**:801

[39] Bernstein CN, Rawsthorne P, Cheang M, Blanchard JF. A population-based case control study of potential risk factors for IBD. The American Journal of Gastroenterology. 2006;**101**(5):993-1002

[40] Timm S, Svanes C, Janson C, et al. Place of upbringing in early childhood as related to inflammatory bowel diseases in adulthood: A population-based cohort study in Northern Europe. European Journal of Epidemiology. 2014;**29**(6):429-437

[41] Bager P, Simonsen J, Nielsen NM, Frisch M. Cesarean section and offspring's risk of inflammatory bowel disease: A national cohort study. Inflammatory Bowel Diseases. 2012;**18**(5):857-862

[42] Castiglione F, Diaferia M, Morace F, et al. Risk factors for inflammatory bowel diseases according to the "hygiene hypothesis": A case-control, multi-centre, prospective study in Southern Italy. Journal of Crohn's & Colitis. 2012;**6**(3):324-329

[43] Ng SC, Tang W, Leong RW, et al. Environmental risk factors in inflammatory bowel disease: A population-based case-control study in Asia-Pacific. Gut. 2015;**64**(7): 1063-1071

[44] Ungaro R, Bernstein CN, Gearry R, et al. Antibiotics associated with increased risk of new-onset Crohn's disease but not ulcerative colitis: A meta-analysis. The American Journal of Gastroenterology. 2014;**109**(11):1728-1738

[45] Shaw SY, Blanchard JF, Bernstein CN. Association between the use of antibiotics in the first year of life and pediatric inflammatory bowel disease. The American Journal of Gastroenterology. 2010;**105**(12):2687-2692

[46] Meyer AM, Ramzan NN, Heigh RI, Leighton JA. Relapse of inflammatory bowel disease associated with use of nonsteroidal anti-inflammatory drugs. Digestive Diseases and Sciences. 2006;**51**(1):168-172

[47] Bernstein CN, Eliakim A, Fedail S, et al. Review Team: World Gastroenterology Organisation Global Guidelines Inflammatory Bowel Disease: Update August 2015. Journal of Clinical Gastroenterology. 2016;**50**(10):803-818

[48] Wang P, Hu J, Ghadermarzi S, et al. Smoking and inflammatory bowel disease: A comparison of China, India, and the USA. Digestive Diseases and Sciences. 2018;**63**(10):2703-2713

[49] Andersson RE, Olaison G, Tysk C, Ekbom A. Appendectomy and protection against ulcerative colitis. The New England Journal of Medicine. 2001;**344**(11):808-814

[50] Andersson RE, Olaison G, Tysk C, Ekbom A. Appendectomy is followed by increased risk of Crohn's disease. Gastroenterology. 2003;**124**(1):40-46

[51] Kikut J, Skonieczna-Żydecka K, Sochaczewska D, Kordek A, Szczuko M. Differences in dietary patterns of adolescent patients with IBD. Nutrients. 2021;**13**(9):3119

[52] Bernstein CN. Psychological stress and depression: Risk factors for IBD? Digestive Diseases. 2016;**34**(1-2):58-63

[53] Graff LA, Walker JR, Bernstein CN. Depression and anxiety in inflammatory bowel disease: A review of comorbidity and management. Inflammatory Bowel Diseases. 2009;**15**:1105-1118

[54] Guthrie E, Jackson J, Shaffer J, et al. Psychological disorder and severity of inflammatory bowel disease predict health-related quality of life in ulcerative colitis and Crohn's disease. The American Journal of Gastroenterology. 2002;**97**:1994-1999

[55] Ananthakrishnan AN, Higuchi LM, Huang ES, et al. Aspirin, nonsteroidal anti-inflammatory drug use, and risk for Crohn disease and ulcerative colitis: A cohort study. Annals of Internal Medicine. 2012;**156**(5):350-359

[56] Kish L, Hotte N, Kaplan GG, et al. Environmental particulate matter induces murine intestinal inflammatory responses and alters the gut microbiome. PLoS One. 2013;**8**(4):e62220

[57] Kaplan GG, Hubbard J, Korzenik J, et al. The inflammatory bowel diseases and ambient air pollution: A novel association. The American Journal of Gastroenterology. 2010;**105**(11):2412-2419

[58] Opstelten JL, Beelen RMJ, Leenders M, et al. Exposure to ambient air pollution and the risk of inflammatory bowel disease: A European Nested Case-Control Study. Digestive Diseases and Sciences. 2016;**61**(10):2963-2971

[59] Eltzschig HK, Carmeliet P. Hypoxia and inflammation. The New England Journal of Medicine. 2011;**364**(7):656-665

[60] Hartmann G, Tschöp M, Fischer R, et al. High altitude increases circulating interleukin-6, interleukin-1 receptor antagonist and C-reactive protein. Cytokine. 2000;**12**(3):246-252

[61] Vermeulen N, Vermeire S, Arijs I, et al. Seroreactivity against glycolytic enzymes in inflammatory bowel disease. Inflammation Bowel Diseases. 2011;**17**(2):557-564

[62] Dulai PS, Buckey JC Jr, Raffals LE, et al. Hyperbaric oxygen therapy is well tolerated and effective for ulcerative colitis patients hospitalized for moderate-severe flares: A phase 2A pilot multi-center, randomized, double-blind, sham-controlled trial. The

American Journal of Gastroenterology. 2018;**113**(10):1516-1523

[63] Hou JK, Abraham B, El-Serag H. Dietary intake and risk of developing inflammatory bowel disease: A systematic review of the literature. The American Journal of Gastroenterology. 2011;**106**(4):563-573

[64] Nie JY, Zhao Q. Beverage consumption and risk of ulcerative colitis: Systematic review and meta-analysis of epidemiological studies. Medicine (Baltimore). 2017;**96**(49):e9070

[65] Wang F, Feng J, Gao Q, et al. Carbohydrate and protein intake and risk of ulcerative colitis: Systematic review and dose-response meta-analysis of epidemiological studies. Clinical Nutrition. 2017;**36**(5):1259-1265

[66] Li F, Liu X, Wang W, Zhang D. Consumption of vegetables and fruit and the risk of inflammatory bowel disease: A meta-analysis. European Journal of Gastroenterology and Hepatology. 2015;**27**(6):623-630

[67] Preda CM, Manuc T, Istratescu D, et al. Environmental factors in Romanian and Belgian patients with inflammatory bowel disease: A Retrospective Comparative Study. Maedica (Bucur). 2019;**14**(3):233-239

[68] Preda CM, Manuc T, Chifulescu A, et al. Diet as an environmental trigger in inflammatory bowel disease: A retrospective comparative study in two European cohorts. Revista Espanola de Enfermedades Digestivas. 2020;**112**(6):440-447

[69] Ge J, Han TJ, Liu J, et al. Meat intake and risk of inflammatory bowel disease: A meta-analysis. The Turkish Journal of Gastroenterology. 2015;**26**(6):492-497

[70] John S, Luben R, Shrestha SS, Welch A, Khaw KT, Hart AR. Dietary n-3 polyunsaturated fatty acids and the aetiology of ulcerative colitis: A UK prospective cohort study. European Journal of Gastroenterology and Hepatology. 2010;**22**(5):602-606

[71] de Silva PS, Olsen A, Christensen J. An association between dietary arachidonic acid, measured in adipose tissue, and ulcerative colitis. Gastroenterology. 2010;**139**(6):1912-1917

[72] Khalili H, Chan SSM, Lochhead P, Ananthakrishnan AN, Hart AR, Chan AT. The role of diet in the aetiopathogenesis of inflammatory bowel disease. Natural Review in Gastroenterology and Hepatology. 2018;**15**(9):525-535

[73] Brown K, DeCoffe D, Molcan E, Gibson DL. Diet-induced dysbiosis of the intestinal microbiota and the effects on immunity and disease. Nutrients. 2012;**4**(8):1095-1119

[74] De Filippo C, Cavalieri D, Di Paola M, et al. Impact of diet in shaping gut microbiota revealed by a comparative study in children from Europe and rural Africa. Proceedings of the National Academy Science U S A. 2010;**107**(33):14691-14696

[75] Sun M, Wu W, Liu Z, Cong Y. Microbiota metabolite short chain fatty acids, GPCR, and inflammatory bowel diseases. Journal of Gastroenterology. 2017;**52**(1):1-8

[76] Agus A, Denizot J, Thévenot J, et al. Western diet induces a shift in microbiota composition enhancing susceptibility to Adherent-Invasive *E. coli* infection and intestinal inflammation. Scientific Reports. 2016;**6**:19032

[77] Machiels K, Joossens M, Sabino J, et al. A decrease of the butyrate-

producing species Roseburiahominis and Faecalibacteriumprausnitzii defines dysbiosis in patients with ulcerative colitis. Gut. 2014;**63**(8):1275-1283

[78] Koleva P, Ketabi A, Valcheva R, Gänzle MG, Dieleman LA. Chemically defined diet alters the protective properties of fructo-oligosaccharides and isomalto-oligosaccharides in HLA-B27 transgenic rats. PLoS One. 2014;**9**(11):e111717

[79] Ananthakrishnan AN, Khalili H, Konijeti GG, et al. Long-term intake of dietary fat and risk of ulcerative colitis and Crohn's disease. Gut. 2014;**63**(5):776-784

[80] Chan SS, Luben R, Olsen A, et al. Association between high dietary intake of the n-3 polyunsaturated fatty acid docosahexaenoic acid and reduced risk of Crohn's disease. Aliment Pharmacological Therapy. 2014;**39**(8):834-842

[81] Chapkin RS, Davidson LA, Ly L, Weeks BR, Lupton JR, McMurray DN. Immunomodulatory effects of (n-3) fatty acids: Putative link to inflammation and colon cancer. The Journal of Nutrition. 2007;**137**(Suppl. 1):200S-204S

[82] Werner T, Wagner SJ, Martínez I, et al. Depletion of luminal iron alters the gut microbiota and prevents Crohn's disease-like ileitis. Gut. 2011;**60**(3):325-333

[83] Sturniolo GC, Di Leo V, Ferronato A, D'Odorico A, D'Incà R. Zinc supplementation tightens "leaky gut" in Crohn's disease. Inflammatory Bowel Diseases. 2001;7(2):94-98

[84] Reich KM, Fedorak RN, Madsen K, Kroeker KI. Vitamin D improves inflammatory bowel disease outcomes: Basic science and clinical review. World Journal of Gastroenterology. 2014;**20**(17):4934-4947

[85] Ruemmele FM. Role of diet in inflammatory bowel disease. Ann NutrMetab. 2016;**68**(Suppl. 1):33-41

[86] Fahoum L, Moscovici A, David S, et al. Digestive fate of dietary carrageenan: evidence of interference with digestive proteolysis and disruption of gut epithelial function. Molecular Nutritional Food Research. 2017;**61**(3). DOI: 10.1002/mnfr.201600545

[87] Chassaing B, Van de Wiele T, De Bodt J, Marzorati M, Gewirtz AT. Dietary emulsifiers directly alter human microbiota composition and gene expression ex vivo potentiating intestinal inflammation. Gut. 2017;**66**(8):1414-1427

[88] Chassaing B, Koren O, Goodrich JK, et al. Dietary emulsifiers impact the mouse gut microbiota promoting colitis and metabolic syndrome. Nature. 2015;**519**(7541):92-96

[89] Kyaw MH, Moshkovska T, Mayberry J. A prospective, randomized, controlled, exploratory study of comprehensive dietary advice in ulcerative colitis: Impact on disease activity and quality of life. European Journal of Gastroenterology and Hepatology. 2014;**26**(8):910-917

[90] Pedersen N, Ankersen DV, Felding M, et al. Low-FODMAP diet reduces irritable bowel symptoms in patients with inflammatory bowel disease. World Journal of Gastroenterology. 2017;**23**(18):3356-3366

[91] Jian L, Anqi H, Gang L, et al. Food exclusion based on IgG antibodies alleviates symptoms in ulcerative colitis:

A Prospective Study. Inflammatory Bowel Diseases. 2018;**24**(9):1918-1925

[92] Lathrop SK, Bloom SM, Rao SM, et al. Peripheral education of the immune system by colonic commensal microbiota. Nature. 2011;**478**(7368):250-254

[93] Morgan XC, Tickle TL, Sokol H, et al. Dysfunction of the intestinal microbiome in inflammatory bowel disease and treatment. Genome Biology. 2012;**13**(9):R79

[94] Nagalingam NA, Lynch SV. Role of the microbiota in inflammatory bowel diseases. Inflammatory Bowel Diseases. 2012;**18**(5):968-984

[95] Spor A, Koren O, Ley R. Unravelling the effects of the environment and host genotype on the gut microbiome. Nature Reviews. Microbiology. 2011;**9**(4):279-290

[96] Duvallet C, Gibbons SM, Gurry T, Irizarry RA, Alm EJ. Meta-analysis of gut microbiome studies identifies disease-specific and shared responses. Nature Communications. 2017;**8**(1):1784

[97] Gevers D, Kugathasan S, Denson LA, et al. The treatment-naive microbiome in new-onset Crohn'sdisease. Cell Host & Microbe. 2014;**15**(3):382-392

[98] Norman JM, Handley SA, Baldridge MT, et al. Disease-specific alterations in the enteric virome in inflammatory bowel disease. Cell. 2015;**160**(3):447-460

[99] Zuo T, Lu XJ, Zhang Y, et al. Gut mucosal virome alterations in ulcerative colitis. Gut. 2019;**68**(7):1169-1179

[100] Qiu X, Ma J, Jiao C, et al. Alterations in the mucosa-associated fungal microbiota in patients with ulcerative colitis. Oncotarget. 2017;**8**(64):107577-107588

[101] Ott SJ, Kühbacher T, Musfeldt M, et al. Fungi and inflammatory bowel diseases: Alterations of composition and diversity. Scandinavian Journal of Gastroenterology. 2008;**43**(7):831-841

[102] Moayyedi P, Surette MG, Kim PT, et al. Fecal microbiota transplantation induces remission in patients with active ulcerative colitis in a randomized controlled trial. Gastroenterology. 2015;**149**(1):102-109

[103] Rossen NG, Fuentes S, van der Spek MJ, et al. Findings from a randomized controlled trial of fecal transplantation for patients with ulcerative colitis. Gastroenterology. 2015;**149**(1):110-118

[104] Costello SP, Hughes PA, Waters O, et al. Effect of fecal microbiota transplantation on 8-week remission in patients with ulcerative colitis: A Randomized Clinical Trial. Journal of the American Medical Association. 2019;**321**(2):156-164

[105] Paramsothy S, Kamm MA, Kaakoush NO, et al. Multidonor intensive faecalmicrobiota transplantation for active ulcerative colitis: A randomised placebo-controlled trial. Lancet. 2017;**389**(10075):1218-1228

[106] Paramsothy S, Nielsen S, Kamm MA, et al. Specific bacteria and metabolites associated with response to fecal microbiota transplantation in patients with ulcerative colitis. Gastroenterology. 2019;**156**(5):1440-1454

[107] Glotzer DJ, Glick ME, Goldman H. Proctitis and colitis following diversion of the fecal stream. Gastroenterology. 1981;**80**(3):438-441

[108] Penders J, Thijs C, Vink C, et al. Factors influencing the composition of the intestinal microbiota in early infancy. Pediatrics. 2006;**118**(2):511-521

[109] Dethlefsen L, Relman DA. Incomplete recovery and individualized responses of the human distal gut microbiota to repeated antibiotic perturbation. Proceedings of the National Academy Science U S A. 2011;**108**(Suppl. 1):4554-4561

[110] Friedrich M, Pohin M, Powrie F. Cytokine networks in the pathophysiology of inflammatory bowel disease. Immunity. 2019;**50**(4):992-1006

[111] Na YR, Stakenborg M, Seok SH, Matteoli G. Macrophages in intestinal inflammation and resolution: A potential therapeutic target in IBD. Natural Reviews in Gastroenterology and Hepatology. 2019;**16**(9):531-543

[112] Graham DB, Luo C, O'Connell DJ, et al. Antigen discovery and specification of immunodominance hierarchies for MHCII-restricted epitopes. Nature Medicine. 2018;**24**(11):1762-1772

[113] Zhou L, Chong MM, Littman DR. Plasticity of CD4+ T cell lineage differentiation. Immunity. 2009;**30**(5):646-655

[114] Reboldi A, Cyster JG. Peyer's patches: Organizing B-cell responses at the intestinal frontier. Immunological Reviews. 2016;**271**(1):230-245

[115] Neurath MF. Cytokines in inflammatory bowel disease. Nature Reviews. Immunology. 2014;**14**(5):329-342

[116] Van Klinken BJ, Van der Wal JW, Einerhand AW, Büller HA, Dekker J. Sulphation and secretion of the predominant secretory human colonic mucin MUC2 in ulcerative colitis. Gut. 1999;**44**(3):387-393

[117] Teng MW, Bowman EP, McElwee JJ, et al. IL-12 and IL-23 cytokines: From discovery to targeted therapies for immune-mediated inflammatory diseases. Nature Medicine. 2015;**21**(7):719-729

[118] Kobayashi T, Okamoto S, Hisamatsu T, et al. IL23 differentially regulates the Th1/Th17 balance in ulcerative colitis and Crohn's disease. Gut. 2008;**57**(12):1682-1689

[119] Nalleweg N, Chiriac MT, Podstawa E, et al. IL-9 and its receptor are predominantly involved in the pathogenesis of UC. Gut. 2015;**64**(5):743-755

[120] Lee JC, Lyons PA, McKinney EF, et al. Gene expression profiling of CD8+ T cells predicts prognosis in patients with Crohn disease and ulcerative colitis. The Journal of Clinical Investigation. 2011;**121**(10):4170-4179

[121] Hepworth MR, Monticelli LA, Fung TC, et al. Innate lymphoid cells regulate CD4+ T-cell responses to intestinal commensal bacteria. Nature. 2013;**498**(7452):113-117

[122] Pantazi E, Powell N. Group 3 ILCs: Peacekeepers or troublemakers? What's your gut telling you?! Frontiers in Immunology. 2019;**10**:676

[123] UK IBD Genetics Consortium, Barrett JC, Lee JC, et al. Genome-wide association study of ulcerative colitis identifies three new susceptibility loci, including the HNF4A region. Nature Genetics. 2009;**41**(12):1330-1334

[124] Rimoldi M, Chieppa M, Salucci V, et al. Intestinal immune homeostasis is regulated by the crosstalk between epithelial cells and dendritic cells. Nature Immunology. 2005;**6**(5):507-514

[125] Ueno A, Ghosh A, Hung D, Li J, Jijon H. Th17 plasticity

and its changes associated with inflammatory bowel disease. World Journal of Gastroenterology. 2015;**21**(43):12283-12295

[126] Park S, Abdi T, Gentry M, Laine L. Histological disease activity as a predictor of clinical relapse among patients with ulcerative colitis: Systematic review and meta-analysis. The American Journal of Gastroenterology. 2016;**111**(12):1692-1701

[127] Dinallo V, Marafini I, Di Fusco D, et al. Neutrophil extracellular traps sustain inflammatory signals in ulcerative colitis. Journal of Crohn's & Colitis. 2019;**13**(6):772-784

[128] Strober W, Fuss IJ. Proinflammatory cytokines in the pathogenesis of inflammatory bowel diseases. Gastroenterology. 2011;**140**(6):1756-1767

[129] de Souza HS, Fiocchi C. Immunopathogenesis of IBD: Current state of the art. Natural Review in Gastroenterology and Hepatology. 2016;**13**(1):13-27

[130] Mann ER, Li X. Intestinal antigen-presenting cells in mucosal immune homeostasis: Crosstalk between dendritic cells, macrophages and B-cells. World Journal of Gastroenterology. 2014;**20**(29):9653-9664

[131] Kmieć Z, Cyman M, Ślebioda TJ. Cells of the innate and adaptive immunity and their interactions in inflammatory bowel disease. Advanced Medical Science. 2017;**62**(1):1-16

[132] Satsangi J, Landers CJ, Welsh KI, Koss K, Targan S, Jewell DP. The presence of anti-neutrophil antibodies reflects clinical and genetic heterogeneity within inflammatory bowel disease. Inflammatory Bowel Diseases. 1998;**4**(1):18-26

[133] West AP, Shadel GS. Mitochondrial DNA in innate immune responses and inflammatory pathology. Natural Review in Immunology. 2017;**17**(6):363-375

[134] Ho GT, Aird RE, Liu B, et al. MDR1 deficiency impairs mitochondrial homeostasis and promotes intestinal inflammation. Mucosal Immunology. 2018;**11**(1):120-130

[135] Boyapati RK, Dorward DA, Tamborska A, et al. Mitochondrial DNA is a pro-inflammatory damage-associated molecular pattern released during active IBD. Inflammatory Bowel Diseases. 2018;**24**(10):2113-2122

[136] Bär F, Bochmann W, Widok A, et al. Mitochondrial gene polymorphisms that protect mice from colitis. Gastroenterology. 2013;**145**(5):1055-1063

[137] Boyapati RK, Tamborska A, Dorward DA, Ho GT. Advances in the understanding of mitochondrial DNA as a pathogenic factor in inflammatory diseases. F1000Res. 2017;**6**:169

[138] Piccinini AM, Midwood KS. DAMPening inflammation by modulating TLR signalling. Mediators of Inflammation. 2010;**2010**:672395

[139] Lamkanfi M, Dixit VM. Mechanisms and functions of inflammasomes. Cell. 2014;**157**(5):1013-1022

[140] Kalla R, Ventham NT, Kennedy NA, Quintana JF, Nimmo ER, Buck AH, et al. MicroRNAs: New players in IBD. Gut. 2015;**64**(3):504-517

[141] Parikh K, Antanaviciute A, Fawkner-Corbett D, et al. Colonic epithelial cell diversity in health and inflammatory bowel disease. Nature. 2019;**567**(7746):49-55

[142] Kinchen J, Chen HH, Parikh K, et al. Structural remodeling of the human

colonic mesenchyme in inflammatory bowel disease. Cell. 2018;**175**(2):370-386

[143] West NR, Hegazy AN, Owens BMJ, et al. Oncostatin M drives intestinal inflammation and predicts response to tumor necrosis factor-neutralizing therapy in patients with inflammatory bowel disease. Nature Medicine. 2017;**23**(5):579-589

Chapter 2

Platelets in Ulcerative Colitis: From Pathophysiology to Therapy

Stanko Petrovic, Slobodan Obradovic, Marijana Petrovic and Nemanja Rancic

Abstract

Based on the role of platelets in inflammation and hemostasis it has been assumed that antiplatelet therapy could be beneficial for patients suffering from ulcerative colitis. Platelets present a link between inflammation and coagulation. They have more than 300 active mediators stored in their granules. Upon activation, platelet degranulate and release a lot of microparticles and mediators and interact with other immune and non-immune cells thereby amplifying inflammation. The most important parameters of platelet activation are P-selectin and CD40 ligand expressed on their surface upon activation, and their soluble forms presented in blood. Today, we have potent anti-platelet drugs that can inhibit platelet activation and degranulation, and thereby reduce inflammation. The most important drugs are P2Y12 receptor antagonists such as ticagrelor and clopidogrel and glycoprotein IIbIIIa inhibitors. Ticagrelor is an active drug and besides antiplatelet activity, it has bactericidal activity against Gram-positive strains and *Clostridium difficile*. Clopidogrel is a prodrug with less anti-inflammatory effect than ticagrelor and no proven bactericidal activity. Glycoprotein IIbIIIa inhibitors are very potent in reducing platelet aggregation but have lower anti-inflammatory potential than ticagrelor and clopidogrel.

Keywords: ulcerative colitis, platelets, antiplatelet therapy, P-selectin, CD40 ligand, ticagrelor, clopidogrel, glycoprotein inhibitors

1. Introduction

Ulcerative colitis (UC) is a chronic disease resulting not only from the abnormal immune response but also from the activation of non-immune cells. Both, immune and non-immune cells are inducing inflammation that causes tissue injury [1, 2]. Platelets (Plt) are now recognized as proinflammatory cells, and aside from their primary role in a hemostasis they also enhance inflammation. The hypercoagulable state exists in the UC patients. Inflammation activates coagulation and coagulation amplifies inflammation [3, 4]. Platelets are unique cells without nucleus that have an important role in hemostasis and thrombosis, with a 5–9-day life span. Platelets have four granule types with stored numerous biologically active substances, such as platelet factor 4, fibrinogen, Von Willebrand factor (vWF), protein S, histamine, prostaglandin E2, platelet growth factor, thromboxane A2, transforming growth factor-beta, coagulation factors, angiogenic and growth factors, β-thromboglobulin, P-selectin (Psel), chemokines, regulated upon activation, normal T cell expressed and presumably secreted (RANTES), monocyte chemotactic protein-1, interleukin (IL) 8 (IL-8), IL-1β, IL-7 [5, 6]. Platelets can interact with many different cells and contribute to vascular inflammation [7]. Platelet factor 4 and β-thromboglobulin are exclusively released from Plt and are increased in the serum of the patients with active UC [8]. Platelet activation is of utmost importance for Plt functioning and is a result of Plt interaction with numerous active molecules. The first step is adhesion to the subendothelial matrix. After that Plt change their shape, resulting in pseudopodia formation [9]. Platelet activation, in the UC patients, takes place in mesenteric microcirculation after exposure to subendothelial collagen, adenosine diphosphate (ADP), arachidonic acid, Plt activating factor, thrombin, fibrinogen, and cytokines from other cells. Upon Plt activation, they degranulate and release a lot of Plt-derived microparticles (PDMP) and preformed mediators and interact with other immune and non-immune cells [10]. The PDMP represent 70–90% of all human cell-derived microparticles and have high procoagulant (due to tissue factor) and proinflammatory potential [11]. They also secrete ADP which in turn bind to the P2Y1 and P2Y12 receptors on the membrane surface of the Plt and amplify initial Plt activation [12].

2. Mechanism of platelets intervention in ulcerative colitis

Upon activation, Plt express receptors on their surface, the most important being glycoprotein IIbIIIA (GPIIbIIIa), CD40 ligand (CD40L), Psel and receptors for cytokines, chemokines, and complement components [13]. A CD40L is a membrane protein, co-stimulatory molecule, presented mostly on the surface of the activated T lymphocyte (T Ly) and activated Plt. Its receptor is CD40, expressed on the surface of the immune cells, endothelial, epithelial cells, Plt, and other mesenchymal cells [14]. After Plt activation, CD40L and Psel are cleaved from the cell surface and secreted in the blood, being called soluble CD40L (sCD40L) and soluble Psel (sPsel). These soluble forms activate other cells, especially endothelial cells, fibroblasts, T Ly, monocyte, neutrophils, and B cells. The CD40/CD40L signaling pathway is a very important pathogenic mechanism in the UC, it amplifies inflammation and activates numerous immune and non-immune cells, including Plt [15, 16]. Platelets are the main source of sCD40L in UC. The number of CD40L positive T Ly and Plt is increased in colonic mucosa [17]. Also, the CD40L-CD40 signaling pathway is responsible for thromboembolic complications in UC patients and inflammation-induced angiogenesis. Platelet dysfunction exists in UC, meaning that Plt are becoming pro-inflammatory cells, and represent a connection between innate and adaptive immunity and between inflammation and coagulation [18].

3. Role of platelets as biomarkers in UC severity

P-selectin is expressed on the membrane surface of the activated Plt and endothelial cells. P-selectin has the most important function in leucocyte (Le) recruitment, mostly in the colonic mucosa [19]. The level of tissue expression of Psel is in strong positive correlation with the level of inflammation in colonic mucosa [20]. In severe inflammation, there is abundant Psel expression in colonic mucosa. Soluble Psel and sCD40L are excellent biomarkers of Plt activation [21].

Abnormalities seen in UC are: elevated Plt count (>450,000 × 10^9/L), reduction in mean Plt volume (MPV), increased platelet distribution width (PDW) value, increased plateletcrit value (PCT), increase in granular content, increased Plt activation and aggregation, hyperreactivity to agonist stimulation, such as ADP and collagen. These abnormalities are mediated by IL-6, are not seen in a healthy person, and are more pronounced in UC than in other inflammatory diseases like rheumatoid arthritis. The MPV and PCT show a negative correlation with disease activity [22–25]. Spontaneous platelet aggregation is observed in more than 30% of UC patients, a phenomenon that is not seen in healthy persons and rarely seen in other inflammatory disorders [26]. Histopathological studies found mesenteric vascular microthrombi to be the first finding in the mucosa of UC patients. Those microthrombi contribute to ischemia. Microthrombi are not found in mesenteric vessels in healthy persons [27]. Activated Plt form aggregates with Le and other Plt, so-called platelet-leukocyte aggregates (PLA) and Plt-Plt aggregates (PPA), via Psel [28]. Platelet-leukocyte aggregate number is increased in serum and colonic tissue of patients with active UC but does not correlate with disease activity, instead, there is a positive correlation with Plt number and serum sPsel concentration. But it is proven that Le within PLA are more active than free Ly or Plt [29]. Platelet-leukocyte aggregate react with endothelial cells, activate them, activate other free Plt and Le. Also, PLA activate endothelial cells more than free cells, leading to increased expression of adhesion molecules thus contributing to inflammation [30]. Increased Plt activation and aggregation, especially spontaneous platelet aggregation, are very much responsible for thrombosis and thromboembolic complications in UC, particularly arterial thrombosis [31, 32].

Platelet to Ly ratio, with cut off value of 175.9 (sensitivity 90.9%; specificity 78.4%; positive likelihood ratio 4.205, 95% confidence interval (95% CI) 2.214–7.894; area under the curve (AUC) 0.897, 95% CI 0.802–0.992) can serve as a biomarker for disease activity in UC, and can help us distinguish UC from healthy controls, that is, to identify UC patients with active disease [33].

We can also use neutrophil to Plt ratio to identify UC patients with active disease, with cut-off point of 14.94 (sensitivity 87.95%; specificity 63.5%) [34].

4. Antiplatelet drugs types

With the developments in medicine, especially pharmacology, we have a lot of antiplatelet drugs, and the number is constantly increasing [35]. The most important antiplatelet drugs are:

1. Thienopyridines represent a group of drugs that blocks ADP-mediated Plt aggregation by blocking the P2Y12 receptor on the Plt membrane surface. After Plt activation, ADP is released from Plt and then binds to P2Y12 on Plt surface and amplifies Plt activation, aggregation, degranulation, and procoagulant activity. Two thienopyridines are most important: clopidogrel and prasugrel. They are prodrugs and require biotransformation to become active. Clopidogrel is used for secondary stroke prevention and after coronary stenting (with aspirin). Prasugrel is used for the prevention of thrombosis after percutaneous coronary interventions [36].

2. Cyclopentyltriazolopyrimidines: ticagrelor. It is an active drug, with a fast onset of action, 30 minutes after ingestion, and it is a reversible P2Y12 receptor antagonist [37].

3. The ADP receptor antagonists: cangrelor. It has a short action time and it is used preoperatively in patients with atherosclerotic disease [38].

4. Aspirin or acetylsalicylic acid is the oldest antiplatelet drug that irreversibly inhibition both cyclooxygenase (COX) 1 and 2 and suppresses the production of prostaglandins and thromboxane. Other non-steroidal anti-inflammatory drugs inhibit COX-1 and Plt function, but their effect is short and reversible [39].

5. Phosphodiesterase inhibitors: dipyridamole that reversibly inactivates platelet cyclic adenosine monophosphate (cAMP)-phosphodiesterase thus increasing cAMP and decreasing Plt activity. Cilostazol is a selective inhibitor of phosphodiesterase type 3 leading to accumulation of cAMP and inhibition of Plt aggregation. It is used for treating peripheral vascular disease [40].

6. GP IIb/IIIa antagonists are anti-Plt agents that block binding GP IIb/IIIa to fibrinogen and inhibit Plt aggregation. Three agents are now being used: abciximab (monoclonal antibody), and two smaller molecule drugs tirofiban and eptifibatide [41].

7. Protease-activated receptor-1 (PAR-1) antagonists: a new class of drugs. Vorapaxar inhibits thrombin-related platelet aggregation [42].

They are used to prevent or treat arterial thrombosis.

The most important indications are: acute coronary syndrome, after the percutaneous coronary intervention (PCI) with stenting, acute ischemic stroke, after percutaneous intervention of peripheral arterial disease, stable angina, and primary prevention of coronary artery disease [43].

Not all anti-Plt agents are the same. Some of them affect mostly Plt aggregation, and some of them affect Plt aggregation and degranulation. The most significant contraindication for anti-Plt agents is active bleeding [44].

The most important antiplatelet drugs with the possibility to be used in UC are clopidogrel, ticagrelor, and GP inhibitors.

Clopidogrel is a prodrug, has 50% bioavailability. After biotransformation in the liver, its active metabolite binds to P2Y12 on the Plt surface and irreversibly inhibits ADP-mediated Plt aggregation and Plt activity. Due to the necessity of the liver biotransformation of clopidogrel by cytochrome P450 (CYP) enzymes CYP3A4/3A5, there is potential for drug interactions and therapeutic failure. Some genetic alterations in the CYP2C19 gene can lead to a low Plt response to clopidogrel [45].

Ticagrelor is an orally active drug. It is a reversible antagonist of P2Y12 receptor on surface Plt membrane that inhibits ADP induced Plt aggregation. It is given twice daily. After ingestion, maximal Plt inhibition was measured at 2–4 hours. It almost completely inhibits Plt aggregation. It has faster and more profound action on Plt inhibition than clopidogrel. Its half-life is 7 hours. After P2Y12 inhibition there is decreased Plt degranulation and decreased releasing of bioactive mediators from Plt, and low expression of Psel and CD40L on Plt surface. Ultimately it leads to reduced generation of PLA and PPA which is considered to be the major mechanism responsible for anti-inflammatory effect. It also inhibits the reuptake of adenosine which leads to its accumulation in the extracellular matrix. Major adverse events are bleeding, dyspnea and bradycardia [46].

Glycoprotein inhibitors compete with fibrinogen and VWF for binding to GPIIbIIIa, which represent the final step in Plt aggregation. They are very potent inhibitors of Plt aggregation. Three GP inhibitors are approved in clinical use: abciximab, eptifibatide, and tirofiban. The route of administration for all three drugs is intravenous. Major adverse events are bleeding and thrombocytopenia. They are very potent in inhibiting Plt aggregation but do not have a potent anti-inflammatory effect [47].

5. The role of antiplatelet drugs in the pathogenesis of UC

Antiplatelet therapy is not a part of standard therapy for treating UC patients, but growing evidence suggest that it is safe in UC and might be useful addition to the standard therapy. I will summarize published results.

This chapter is based on an evaluation of antiplatelet therapy in patients with UC. We defined key questions as our literature searching algorithm. We searched literature from PubMed according to the adequate MESH terms ("ulcerative colitis," "platelets," "antiplatelet therapy," "P-selectin," "CD40 ligand," "ticagrelor," "clopidogrel," and "glycoprotein inhibitors") for the period from 2000 to the present.

5.1 Antiplatelet agents'-ticagrelor and eptifibatide-safety in experimental colitis in mice

The authors conducted an animal study about the usage of antiplatelet agents—ticagrelor and eptifibatide in mice. Forty C57BL/6 mice (inbred females, age: 2–3 months, and average body mass: 20–24 g) were used. The bodyweight of mice was measured every day. Mice were observed for stool consistency and rectal bleeding on a daily basis so that disease activity index (DAI) could be calculated daily as the sum of the weight loss score, the diarrheal score, and the hematochezia score based on the method used by Friedman et al., as shown in **Table 1**. The DAI was used to assess the severity of colitis [48].

Colitis was induced in 30 mice by 5-day drinking water with 3.5% dextran sulfate sodium (DSS) (average molecular weight within the range of 35,000–55,000). All mice developed DSS colitis. After 5 days, DSS-induced mice were divided into three experimental groups, 10 each. The first (I) group, the DSS control group, received no intervention during the subsequent 5 days treatment period. The second (II) group, the ticagrelor treatment (PO) group, received 1 mg (in 0.5 mL) dosages per day of

	DAI score				
	0	1	2	3	4
Weight loss	0%	1–5%	6–10%	11–20%	>20%
Stoll consistency	Well-formed pellets		Semi-formed pellets		Liquid stools
Rectal bleeding	Hemoccult negative		Hemoccult positive		Gross bleeding

Table 1.
Disease activity index (DAI).

Brilinta® via gastric tube. The third (III) group, the eptifibatide treatment (IP) group, received 150 µg (in 0.2 mL) dosages per day of Integrilin® via intraperitoneal injection. Group of mice (n = 10), experimental control (K) group, received water without DSS during the 5 days period.

The primary outcome was bleeding, and the secondary outcomes were changes in platelet count, hemoglobin (Hgb) level, and hematocrit (HCT) level. Complete blood counts were determined for each group at baseline (day 0: before treatment; DSS1, PO1, and IP1 subgroups) and at 1 day after the last dose (day 5; DSS2, PO2, and IP2 subgroups). On day 5, all surviving mice were sacrificed, and an autopsy was performed. The Plt aggregation was measured using a multiplate Plt function analyzer with adenosine diphosphate and thrombin receptor-activating peptide.

Platelet aggregation was measured at baseline, after 2 h, and 24 h of ticagrelor and eptifibatide therapy. An autopsy showed signs of colitis and there was no evidence of recent bleeding in the liver, spleen, central nervous system, or serous cavities of any of the antiplatelet treatment groups. Histological findings of colonic mucosa in all three experimental groups after autopsy were that DSS2, PO2, and IP2 showed mild inflammation and ulceration.

Maximum weight loss was below 15% in all three experimental groups. Hematochezia was observed in all three experimental groups as blood around the anus and present in the sawdust or as hemoccult positive. Blood was seen from the fourth day of the experiment in all three experimental groups.

The DAI score was not significantly different between the three experimental groups (Kruskal-Wallis test; p = 0.925).

Significantly lower levels of Hgb and HCT were found in all three experimental groups (PO1, DSS1, PO1, and IP1 vs. control; Kruskal-Wallis test: p = 0.007 and p = 0.002, respectively) (**Figures 1** and **2**). However, the Plt count was not significantly different between any of the DSS groups and the control group (Kruskal-Wallis test: p = 0.640) (**Figure 3**). There were no significant differences in the drug-related changes in the Hgb, HCT, and Plt levels of the three DSS groups according to the two drugs administered (baseline vs. end of treatment; Kruskal-Wallis test: HGB, p = 0.369; HCT, p = 0.104; and Plt, p = 0.307) (**Figures 4–6**).

The authors concluded that administering eptifibatide and ticagrelor to DSS colitis mice did not cause serious adverse events. There was no significant decrease in Plt

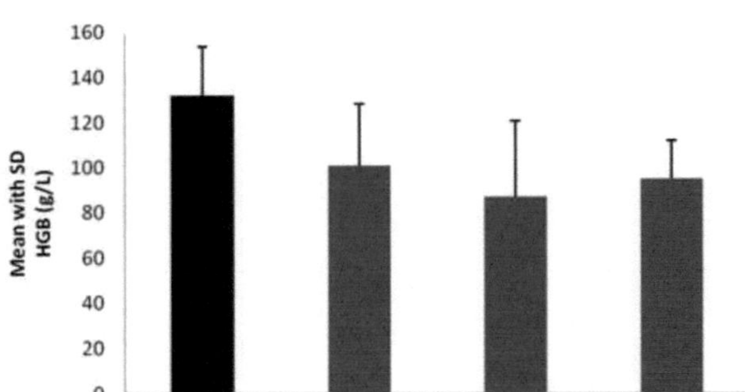

	K	DSS1	PO1	IP1
■ Mean HGB	132.1	101.0	87.0	94.7

Figure 1.
Hemoglobin (Hgb) values before initiation of antiplatelet drug administration. Data are presented as mean ± SD. Groups DSS1, IP1, and PO1 represent DSS colitis mice before administration of drugs; K represents the experimental control group. DSS, dextran sulfate sodium; IP, eptifibatide treatment; PO, ticagrelor treatment.

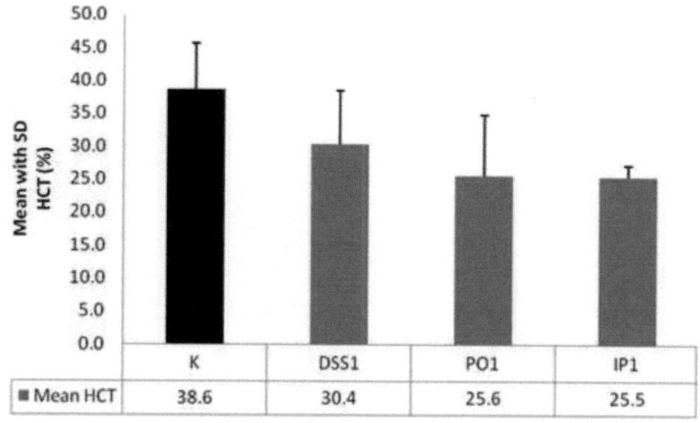

Figure 2.
Hematocrit (HCT) values before initiation of antiplatelet drug administration. Data are presented as mean ± SD. Groups DSS1, IP1, and PO1 represent DSS colitis mice before administration of drugs; K represents the experimental control group. DSS, dextran sulfate sodium; IP, eptifibatide treatment; PO, ticagrelor treatment (Kruskal-Wallis test: p = 0.002).

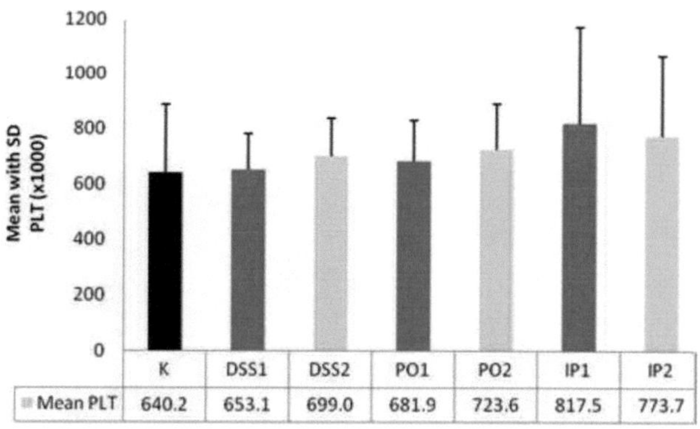

Figure 3.
Platelet (PLT) count for all groups. Data are presented as mean ± SD. Groups DSS1, IP1, and PO1 represent DSS colitis mice before administration of drugs; K represents the experimental control group. Groups DSS2, IP2, and PO2 represent DSS colitis mice after administration of drugs. DSS, dextran sulfate sodium; IP, eptifibatide treatment; PO, ticagrelor treatment (Kruskal-Wallis test: p = 0.640).

count or Hgb and HCT levels, and autopsy found no bleeding into the liver, spleen, serous cavities or intracranially. These observations support the potential use of antiplatelet therapy for treating UC in humans as an addition to the standard therapy. Ticagrelor could be used in the moderate form of UC and eptifibatide in the severe form, together with standard therapy.

5.2 Evaluation of anti-inflammatory effect of anti-platelet agent-clopidogrel in experimentally induced inflammatory bowel disease

The goal of this research was to evaluate the anti-inflammatory effect of clopidogrel on an animal model for Crohn's disease (TNBS model) and ulcerative colitis (oxazolone induced) in rats. Rats were weighing 150–200 g and were housed in standard conditions, on a standard diet and water ad libitum. Ulcerative colitis was induced by intrarectal administration of oxazolone on first day. Rats were divided into four groups, each consisting of six animals: **Control** group (healthy rats),

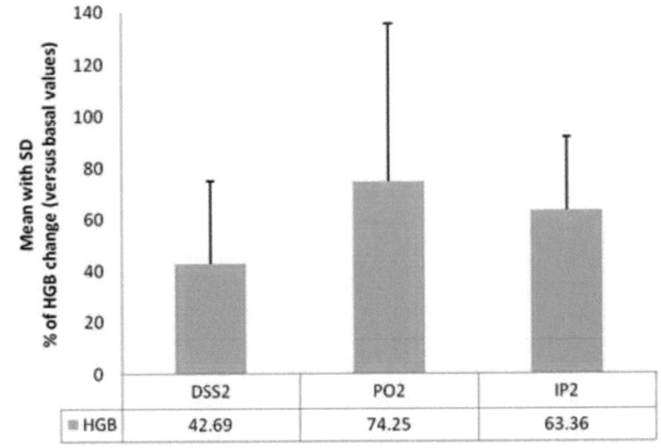

Figure 4.
Percent change in values of hemoglobin (Hgb) relative to basal values. Groups DSS2, IP2, and PO2 represent DSS colitis mice after administration of drugs. DSS, dextran sulfate sodium; IP, eptifibatide treatment; PO, ticagrelor treatment (Kruskal-Wallis test: HGB, p = 0.369).

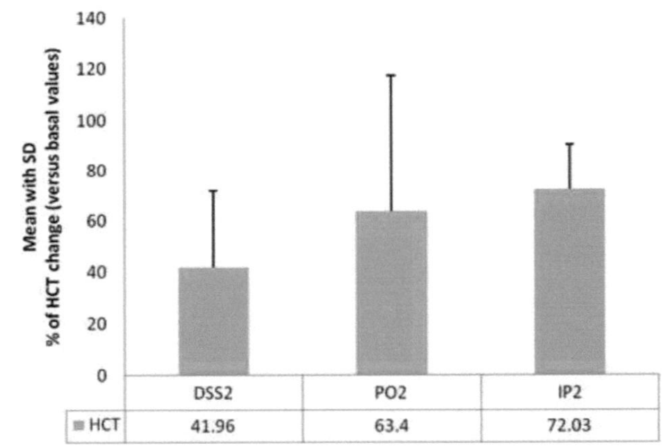

Figure 5.
Percent change in values of hematocrit (HCT) relative to basal values. Groups DSS2, IP2, and PO2 represent DSS colitis mice after administration of drugs. DSS, dextran sulfate sodium; IP, eptifibatide treatment; PO, ticagrelor treatment (Kruskal-Wallis test: HCT, p = 0.104).

Oxazolone group (induced UC without treatment), **Standard** group (oxazolone + sulfasalazine for the next 21 days), and **Test** group (oxazolone + clopidogrel per os for the next 21 days). At regular time intervals percentage change in body weight, colon mucosal damage index (CMDI), DAI, and myeloperoxidase (MPO) activity were measured. The CMDI, DAI, and MPO were used to assess inflammatory changes in colonic mucosa. It was shown that the test group resolved symptoms and significantly reduced MPO activity, DAI, and CMDI, better than other groups [49].

5.3 Acetylsalicylic acid reduces the severity of dextran sodium sulfate-induced colitis and increases the formation of anti-inflammatory lipid mediators

The goal of this study was to evaluate the effect of acetylsalicylic acid (ASA) on DSS colitis in mice. Female C57BL/6 mice, average body weight 19–21 g, were divided into three groups: **Control group**, **another group** receiving 3% DSS and no treatment

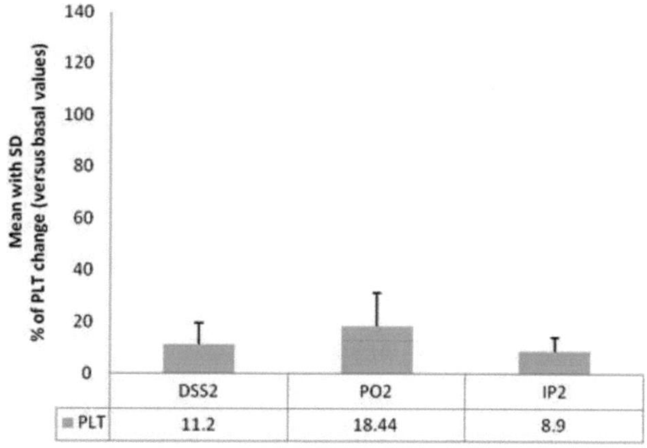

Figure 6.
Percent change in values of platelets (PLT) relative to basal values. Groups DSS2, IP2, and PO2 represent DSS colitis mice after administration of drugs. DSS, dextran sulfate sodium; IP, eptifibatide treatment; PO, ticagrelor treatment (Kruskal-Wallis test: PLT, p = 0.307).

and **ASA** group, receiving 3% DSS and daily intraperitoneal ASA for 5 days. Bodyweight, occult blood in stool samples, histological evaluation of the distal colon, and magnetic resonance imaging (MRI) were measured to evaluate colitis severity. The authors concluded that DSS colitis can be alleviated by ASA [50].

5.4 CD40-CD40 ligand mediates the recruitment of leukocytes and platelets in the inflamed murine colon

The aim of this study was to evaluate the role of the CD40-CD40L signaling pathway in intestinal inflammation in DSS colitis in mice and the anti-inflammatory effect of Trapidil (triazolopyrimidine) on intestinal inflammation. Trapidil is an antagonist of platelet-derived growth factor and it was developed to inhibit the response of monocytes to CD40L. They found a 10-fold increase in CD40 expression in endothelial cells in the colon (an important result of CD40-CD40L signaling pathway), increased recruitment of Plt and leukocytes in colonic venules due to CD40-CD40L pathway and significant inhibition of CD40-CD40L signaling pathway with Trapidil [51].

5.5 The role of P-selectin in experimental colitis as determined by antibody immunoblockade and genetically deficient mice

The objective of this study was to evaluate the role of Psel on leukocyte recruitment and the effect of its blockade with an anti-P-sel antibody. They induced DSS colitis in wild type and P-selectin−/− C57BL/6 J mice. Disease activity index, plasma IL-6, length of colon and rectum, histological damage of the colon, and MPO activity of the distal colon were evaluated. Leukocyte-endothelial interaction in colonic venules was assessed using intravital microscopy. Vascular cell adhesion protein 1 (VCAM-1) and intercellular adhesion molecule 1 expression on endothelial cells and expression of very large antigen-4 integrin on circulating leukocytes were obtained. They found that Psel has an important role in intestinal inflammation in DSS colitis. Its blockade or genetic deficiency offers protection against DSS colitis. They also found that treatment of DSS colitis with Psel antibody was very potent in reducing

DAI, MPO activity, and leukocyte adhesion. The VCAM-1 over-expression in the colon and extracolonic organs and increased level of IL-6 in circulation were observed in P-selectin−/− mice, but not in mice treated with anti-P-sel antibodies. The conclusion was that Psel is a key molecule for the development of DSS colitis and that Psel antibodies administration or genetic deficiency offers protection against DSS colitis by diminishing leukocyte recruitment in the colon [52].

5.6 Daily aspirin use does not impact clinical outcomes in patients with inflammatory bowel disease

It was a retrospective analysis of 174 patients with pre-existing inflammatory bowel disease, who were taking aspirin, due to cardiac comorbidity, for at least 18 months and did not differ in age, gender, disease duration, smoking status, medication usage, or baseline C-reactive protein. They were looking for the connection between aspirin and inflammatory bowel disease (IBD) related hospitalization/surgery/corticosteroid required during the period of follow-up. Their results indicate that aspirin use did not have a clinical impact on IBD patients [53].

6. The role of antiplatelet drugs in the treatment of UC

A retrospective analysis of 36 patients with pre-existing IBD (test group), who started on combination therapy of aspirin and clopidogrel for at least 6 months, due to PCI for coronary artery disease. There was a control group with IBD matched for gender and age, not taking antiplatelet therapy. They found no change in frequency of IBD exacerbations between groups, after the initiation of the aspirin and clopidogrel in the test group [54].

6.1 Antibacterial activity of ticagrelor in conventional antiplatelet dosages against antibiotic-resistant Gram-positive bacteria

After analysis of the PLATO study, the question was raised whether ticagrelor has antibacterial activity in standard anti Plt dosages against Gram-positive bacteria because patients treated with ticagrelor had a lower risk of infection-related death than patients treated with clopidogrel. Authors proved that in vitro ticagrelor has bactericidal activity against all Gram-positive strains tested, including drug-resistant strains glycopeptide intermediate *Staphylococcus aureus*, methicillin-resistant *Staphylococcus epidermidis*, methicillin-resistant *S. aureus*, and vancomycin-resistant *Enterococcus faecalis*. These bactericidal concentrations are not reached in the systemic circulation but might be reached at the infection site probably by drug accumulation [55].

6.2 Repurposing a platelet aggregation inhibitor ticagrelor as an antimicrobial against Clostridioides difficile

The author tested the antimicrobial activity of ticagrelor against different types of *Clostridium difficile* (C. diff) in vitro. They found that ticagrelor has minimal inhibitory concentration (MIC) 20–40 μg/ml for all types of C. diff. Ticagrelor had a more rapid killing profile compared to metronidazole and vancomycin, and also inhibited biofilm formation, which is very important for the pathogenicity of C. diff infection.

Ticagrelor effectively reduced spore germination of C. diff, caused membrane disruption in C. diff and had an additive effect on metronidazole and vancomycin [56].

7. Conclusion

The exact pathophysiology of ulcerative colitis is unknown. Except immune cells, it is important to take platelet function into the consideration so we could improve the response rate to the standard therapy in ulcerative colitis patients. Antiplatelet therapy is still not a part of the therapeutic armamentarium for this disease. We have increasing evidence that raises the possibility of using antiplatelet therapy in humans with ulcerative colitis. Antiplatelet therapy in UC is safe and it seems that ticagrelor could be the drug of the first choice.

Conflict of interest

The authors declare no conflict of interest.

Acronyms and abbreviations

ASA	acetylsalicylic acid
ADP	adenosine diphosphate
AUC	area under the curve
CD40L	CD40 ligand
C. diff	*Clostridium difficile*
CMDI	colon mucosal damage index
cAMP	cyclic adenosine monophosphate
COX	cyclooxygenase
CYP	cytochrome P450
DSS	dextran sulfate sodium
DAI	disease activity index
GPIIbIIIa	glycoprotein IIbIIIA
HCT	hematocrit
Hgb	hemoglobin
IBD	inflammatory bowel disease
IL	interleukin
Le	leucocyte
MRI	magnetic resonance imaging
MPV	mean Plt volume
MIC	minimal inhibitory concentration
MPO	myeloperoxidase
PCT	plateletcrit
PCI	percutaneous coronary intervention
PDW	platelet distribution width
PLA	platelet-leukocyte aggregates
Plt	platelets
Psel	P-selectin
PDMP	Plt derived microparticles

PPA	Plt-Plt aggregates
PAR-1	protease-activated receptor-1
RANTES	regulated upon activation, normal T cell expressed and presumably secreted
sCD40L	soluble CD40L
sPsel	soluble Psel
T Ly	T lymphocyte
UC	ulcerative colitis
VCAM-1	vascular cell adhesion protein 1
vWF	Von Willebrand factor
95% CI	95% confidence interval

Author details

Stanko Petrovic*, Slobodan Obradovic, Marijana Petrovic and Nemanja Rancic
Military Medical Academy, Belgrade, Serbia

*Address all correspondence to: stanko53p@gmail.com

References

[1] Danese S. Nonimmune cells in inflammatory bowel disease: From victim to villain. Trends in Immunology. 2008;**29**:555-564. DOI: 10.1016/j.it.2008.07.009

[2] Danese S, Scaldaferri F, Papa A, Pola R, Sans M, Gasbarrini G, et al. Platelets: New players in the mucosal scenario of inflammatory bowel disease. European Review for Medical and Pharmacological Sciences. 2004;**8**:193-198

[3] Yoshida H, Granger DN. Inflammatory bowel disease: A paradigm for the link between coagulation and inflammation. Inflammatory Bowel Diseases. 2009;**15**:1245-1255. DOI: 10.1002/ibd.20896

[4] Voudoukis E, Karmiris K, Koutroubakis IE. Multipotent role of platelets in inflammatory bowel diseases: A clinical approach. World Journal of Gastroenterology. 2014;**20**:3180-3190. DOI: 10.3748/wjg.v20.i12.3180

[5] Jurk K, Kehrel BE. Platelets: Physiology and biochemistry. Seminars in Thrombosis and Hemostasis. 2005;**31**: 381-392. DOI: 10.1055/s-2005-916671

[6] Maouia A, Rebetz J, Kapur R, Semple JW. The immune nature of platelets revisited. Transfusion Medicine Reviews. 2020;**34**:209-220. DOI: 10.1016/j.tmrv.2020.09.005

[7] Ware JA, Heistad DD. Seminars in medicine of the Beth Israel Hospital, Boston. Platelet-endothelium interactions. The New England Journal of Medicine. 1993;**328**:628-635. DOI: 10.1056/NEJM199303043280907

[8] Vrij AA, Rijken J, Van Wersch JW, Stockbrügger RW. Platelet factor 4 and beta-thromboglobulin in inflammatory bowel disease and giant cell arteritis. European Journal of Clinical Investigation. 2000;**30**:188-194. DOI: 10.1046/j.1365-2362.2000.00616.x

[9] Nieswandt B, Pleines I, Bender M. Platelet adhesion and activation mechanisms in arterial thrombosis and ischaemic stroke. Journal of Thrombosis and Haemostasis. 2011;**9**(Suppl 1):92-104. DOI: 10.1111/j.1538-7836.2011.04361.x

[10] Andoh A, Tsujikawa T, Hata K, Araki Y, Kitoh K, Sasaki M, et al. Elevated circulating plateletderived microparticles in patients with active inflammatory bowel disease. The American Journal of Gastroenterology. 2005;**100**:2042-2048. DOI: 10.1111/j.1572-0241.2005.50381.x

[11] Horstman LL, Ahn YS. Platelet microparticles: A wide-angle perspective. Critical Reviews in Oncology/Hematology. 1999;**30**:111-142. DOI: 10.1016/S1040-8428(98)00044-4

[12] Remijn JA, Wu YP, Jeninga EH, Ijsseldijk MJ, van Willigen G, de Groot PG, et al. Role of ADP receptor P2Y(12) in platelet adhesion and thrombus formation in flowing blood. Arteriosclerosis, Thrombosis, and Vascular Biology. 2002;**22**:686-691. DOI: 10.1161/01.atv.0000012805.49079.23

[13] Scaldaferri F, Lancellotti S, Pizzoferrato M, De Cristofaro R. Haemostatic system in inflammatory bowel diseases: New players in gut inflammation. World Journal of Gastroenterology. 2011;**17**:594-608. DOI: 10.3748/wjg.v17.i5.594

[14] Senhaji N, Kojok K, Darif Y, Fadainia C, Zaid Y. The contribution

of CD40/CD40L axis in inflammatory bowel disease: An update. Frontiers in Immunology. 2015;**6**:529. DOI: 10.3389/fimmu.2015.00529

[15] Göke M, Hoffmann JC, Evers J, Krüger H, Manns MP. Elevated serum concentrations of soluble selectin and immunoglobulin type adhesion molecules in patients with inflammatory bowel disease. Journal of Gastroenterology. 1997;**32**:480-486. DOI: 10.1007/BF02934086

[16] Danese S, Sans M, Fiocchi C. The CD40/CD40L costimulatory pathway in inflammatory bowel disease. Gut. 2004;**53**:1035-1043. DOI: 10.1136/gut.2003.026278

[17] Danese S, Katz JA, Saibeni S, Papa A, Gasbarrini A, Vecchi M, et al. Activated platelets are the source of elevated levels of soluble CD40 ligand in the circulation of inflammatory bowel disease patients. Gut. 2003;**52**:1435-1441. DOI: 10.1136/gut.52.10.1435

[18] Koutroubakis IE, Theodoropoulou A, Xidakis C, Sfiridaki A, Notas G, Kolios G, et al. Association between enhanced soluble CD40 ligand and prothrombotic state in inflammatory bowel disease. European Journal of Gastroenterology & Hepatology. 2004;**16**:1147-1152. DOI: 10.1097/00042737-200411000-00011

[19] Fägerstam JP, Whiss PA, Ström M, Andersson RG. Expression of platelet P-selectin and detection of soluble P-selectin, NPY and RANTES in patients with inflammatory bowel disease. Inflammation Research. 2000;**49**:466-472. DOI: 10.1007/s000110050618

[20] Schürmann GM, Bishop AE, Facer P, Vecchio M, Lee JC, Rampton DS, et al. Increased expression of cell adhesion molecule P-selectin in active inflammatory bowel disease. Gut. 1995;**36**:411-418. DOI: 10.1136/gut.36.3.411

[21] Matowicka-Karna J. Markers of inflammation, activation of blood platelets and coagulation disorders in inflammatory bowel diseases. Postepy Higieny i Medycyny Doświadczalnej (Online). 2016;**70**:305-312. DOI: 10.5604/17322693.1199305

[22] Collins CE, Rampton DS. Platelet dysfunction: A new dimension in inflammatory bowel disease. Gut. 1995;**36**:5-8. DOI: 10.1136/gut.36.1.5

[23] Senchenkova EY, Komoto S, Russell J, Almeida-Paula LD, Yan LS, Zhang S, et al. Interleukin-6 mediates the platelet abnormalities and thrombogenesis associated with experimental colitis. The American Journal of Pathology. 2013;**183**:173-181. DOI: 10.1016/j.ajpath.2013.03.014

[24] Cioffi M, Rosa AD, Serao R, Picone I, Vietri MT. Laboratory markers in ulcerative colitis: Current insights and future advances. World Journal of Gastrointestinal Pathophysiology. 2015;**6**:13-22. DOI: 10.4291/wjgp.v6.i1.13

[25] Webberley MJ, Hart MT, Melikian V. Thromboembolism in inflammatory bowel disease: Role of platelets. Gut. 1993;**34**:247-251. DOI: 10.1136/gut.34.2.247

[26] Danese S, Motte Cd Cde L, Fiocchi C. Platelets in inflammatory bowel disease: Clinical, pathogenic, and therapeutic implications. The American Journal of Gastroenterology. 2004;**99**:938-945. DOI: 10.1111/j.1572-0241.2004.04129.x

[27] Dhillon AP, Anthony A, Sim R, Wakefield AJ, Sankey EA, Hudson M, et al. Mucosal capillary thrombi in rectal biopsies. Histopathology. 1992;**21**:127-133. DOI: 10.1111/j.1365-2559.1992.tb00360.x

[28] Celi A, Pellegrini G, Lorenzet R, De Blasi A, Ready N, Furie BC, et al. P-selectin induces the expression of tissue factor on monocytes. Proceedings of the National Academy of Sciences of the United States of America. 1994;**91**:8767-8771. DOI: 10.1073/pnas.91.19.8767

[29] Peters MJ, Dixon G, Kotowicz KT, Hatch DJ, Heyderman RS, Klein NJ. Circulating platelet-neutrophil complexes represent a subpopulation of activated neutrophils primed for adhesion, phagocytosis and intracellular killing. British Journal of Haematology. 1999;**106**:391-399. DOI: 10.1046/j.1365-2141.1999.01553.x

[30] Tekelioğlu Y, Uzun H. Circulating platelet-leukocyte aggregates in patients with inflammatory bowel disease. Journal of the Chinese Medical Association. 2013;**76**:182-185. DOI: 10.1016/j.jcma.2012.12.015. Erratum in: J Chin Med Assoc. 2013;76:657. Güçer, Hasan [removed]

[31] Irving PM, Macey MG, Shah U, Webb L, Langmead L, Rampton DS. Formation of platelet-leukocyte aggregates in inflammatory bowel disease. Inflammatory Bowel Diseases. 2004;**10**:361-372. DOI: 10.1097/00054725-200407000-00007

[32] Zezos P, Kouklakis G, Saibil F. Inflammatory bowel disease and thromboembolism. World Journal of Gastroenterology. 2014;**20**:13863-13878. DOI: 10.3748/wjg.v20.i38.13863

[33] Jeong Y, Jeon SR, Kim HG, Moon JR, Lee TH, Jang JY, et al. The role of platelet to lymphocyte ratio and neutrophil to lymphocyte ratio in ulcerative colitis. Intestinal Research. 2021;**19**:62-70. DOI: 10.5217/ir.2019.09156

[34] Yamamoto-Furusho JK, Mendieta-Escalante EA. Diagnostic utility of the neutrophil-platelet ratio as a novel marker of activity in patients with ulcerative colitis. PLoS One. 2020;**15**:e0231988. DOI: 10.1371/journal.pone.0231988

[35] McFadyen JD, Schaff M, Peter K. Current and future antiplatelet therapies: Emphasis on preserving haemostasis. Nature Reviews. Cardiology. 2018;**15**:181-191. DOI: 10.1038/nrcardio.2017.206

[36] Hashemzadeh M, Goldsberry S, Furukawa M, Khoynezhad A, Movahed MR. ADP receptor-blocker thienopyridines: Chemical structures, mode of action and clinical use. A review. The Journal of Invasive Cardiology. 2009;**21**:406-412

[37] Goffin E, Jacques N, Musumeci L, Nchimi A, Oury C, Lancellotti P, et al. Synthesis of ticagrelor analogues belonging to 1,2,3-triazolo[4,5-d] pyrimidines and study of their antiplatelet and antibacterial activity. European Journal of Medicinal Chemistry. 2020;**208**:112767. DOI: 10.1016/j.ejmech.2020.112767

[38] De Luca L, Steg PG, Bhatt DL, Capodanno D, Angiolillo DJ. Cangrelor: Clinical data, contemporary use, and future perspectives. Journal of the American Heart Association. 2021;**10**:e022125. DOI: 10.1161/JAHA.121.022125

[39] Fuster V, Sweeny JM. Aspirin: A historical and contemporary therapeutic overview. Circulation. 2011;**123**:768-778. DOI: 10.1161/CIRCULATIONAHA.110.963843

[40] Shafiee-Nick R, Afshari AR, Mousavi SH, Rafighdoust A, Askari VR, Mollazadeh H, et al. A comprehensive review on the potential therapeutic benefits of phosphodiesterase inhibitors on cardiovascular diseases. Biomedicine

& Pharmacotherapy. 2017;**94**:541-556. DOI: 10.1016/j.biopha.2017.07.084

[41] Ji X, Hou M. Novel agents for anti-platelet therapy. Journal of Hematology & Oncology. 2011;**4**:44. DOI: 10.1186/1756-8722-4-44

[42] Bhandari B, Mehta B. Vorapaxar, a protease-activated receptor-1 antagonist, a double-edged sword! Recent Advances in Cardiovascular Drug Discovery. 2014;**9**:73-77. DOI: 10.2174/1574890110666150624100815

[43] Thachil J. Antiplatelet therapy—A summary for the general physicians. Clinical Medicine (London, England). 2016;**16**:152-160. DOI: 10.7861/clinmedicine.16-2-152

[44] Pitchford SC. Novel uses for anti-platelet agents as anti-inflammatory drugs. British Journal of Pharmacology. 2007;**152**:987-1002. DOI: 10.1038/sj.bjp.0707364

[45] Jarvis B, Simpson K. Clopidogrel: A review of its use in the prevention of atherothrombosis. Drugs. 2000;**60**:347-377. DOI: 10.2165/00003495-200060020-00012. Erratum in: Drugs. 2001;61:52

[46] Dobesh PP, Oestreich JH. Ticagrelor: Pharmacokinetics, pharmacodynamics, clinical efficacy, and safety. Pharmacotherapy. 2014;**34**:1077-1090. DOI: 10.1002/phar.1477

[47] Stangl PA, Lewis S. Review of currently available GP IIb/IIIa inhibitors and their role in peripheral vascular interventions. Seminars in Interventional Radiology. 2010;**27**:412-421. DOI: 10.1055/s-0030-1267856

[48] Petrovic SS, Vasiljevska MM, Obradovic SD, Tarabar DK, Doder RB, Majstorovic IJ, et al. Antiplatelet agents'-ticagrelol and eptifibatide-safety in experimental colitis in mice. The Turkish Journal of Gastroenterology. 2020;**31**:451-458. DOI: 10.5152/tjg.2020.19454

[49] Patel SH, Rachchh MA, Jadav PD. Evaluation of anti-inflammatory effect of anti-platelet agent-clopidogrel in experimentally induced inflammatory bowel disease. Indian Journal of Pharmacology. 2012;**44**:744-748. DOI: 10.4103/0253-7613.103278

[50] Köhnke T, Gomolka B, Bilal S, Zhou X, Sun Y, Rothe M, et al. Acetylsalicylic acid reduces the severity of dextran sodium sulfate-induced colitis and increases the formation of anti-inflammatory lipid mediators. BioMed Research International. 2013;**2013**:748160. DOI: 10.1155/2013/748160

[51] Vowinkel T, Anthoni C, Wood KC, Stokes KY, Russell J, Gray L, et al. CD40-CD40 ligand mediates the recruitment of leukocytes and platelets in the inflamed murine colon. Gastroenterology. 2007;**132**:955-965. DOI: 10.1053/j.gastro.2006.12.027

[52] Gironella M, Mollà M, Salas A, Soriano A, Sans M, Closa D, et al. The role of P-selectin in experimental colitis as determined by antibody immunoblockade and genetically deficient mice. Journal of Leukocyte Biology. 2002;**72**:56-64

[53] Patel P, Gao G, Gulotta G, Dalal S, Cohen RD, Sakuraba A, et al. Daily aspirin use does not impact clinical outcomes in patients with inflammatory bowel disease. Inflammatory Bowel Diseases. 2021;**27**:236-241. DOI: 10.1093/ibd/izaa060

[54] Vinod J, Vadada D, Fields S, Baiocco P. The effect of anti-platelet therapy on inflammatory bowel

disease. The American Journal of Gastroenterology. 2008;**103**:S432-S433

[55] Lancellotti P, Musumeci L, Jacques N, Servais L, Goffin E, Pirotte B, et al. Antibacterial activity of ticagrelor in conventional antiplatelet dosages against antibiotic-resistant Gram-positive bacteria. JAMA Cardiology. 2019;**4**:596-599. DOI: 10.1001/jamacardio.2019.1189

[56] Phanchana M, Phetruen T, Harnvoravongchai P, Raksat P, Ounjai P, Chankhamhaengdecha S, et al. Repurposing a platelet aggregation inhibitor ticagrelor as an antimicrobial against Clostridioides difficile. Scientific Reports. 2020;**10**:6497. DOI: 10.1038/s41598-020-63199-x

Section 2

Symptomatology

Chapter 3

Complications of Ulcerative Colitis in Children

Sabina Wiecek

Abstract

Inflammatory bowel disease is a group of chronic disorders of the gastrointestinal tract, including Lesniowski-Crohn disease, ulcerative colitis, and indeterminate colitis. The most frequently occurring symptoms in patients with IBD, including ulcerative colitis, involve abdominal discomfort, recurring and often bloody diarrhoea, weight loss, and the resulting anaemia and/or cachexia. Extraintestinal manifestations of ulcerative colitis may precede the diagnosis of inflammatory bowel disease, they may also occur during remission (pyoderma gangrenosum, uveitis, spondylitis, and PSC) or accompany an exacerbation of the disease (erythema nodosum, episcleritis, aphthae, and some forms of peripheral spondyloarthritis). This study focuses on the most common extraintestinal manifestations and complications in ulcerative colitis in paediatric patients.

Keywords: ulcerative colitis, parenteral symptoms, complications, children

1. Introduction

Inflammatory bowel disease is a group of chronic disorders of the gastrointestinal tract, including Lesniowski-Crohn disease, ulcerative colitis, and indeterminate colitis. The course of these disorders is characterised by alternating periods of remission, which may last even a few years, and exacerbation. Chronic inflammatory bowel diseases develop as a result of coexisting genetic, immunological and environmental factors, and the immune system, which is linked to the digestive system and constitutes a vast proportion of the whole defence mechanism of our body. Among the most frequently occurring symptoms in patients with IBD, including ulcerative colitis, are abdominal discomfort, recurring and often bloody diarrhoea, weight loss, and the resulting anaemia and/or cachexia. The aspects of extraintestinal symptoms of inflammatory bowel diseases are not discussed often, and yet in as many as 40–50% of patients, at least one extraintestinal manifestation of IBD occurs with even 25% of patients reporting two or more symptoms not related to the digestive system. The causes of the occurrence of extraintestinal symptoms in the course of ulcerative colitis have been widely discussed. Increased permeability of the intestinal wall allows for the contents of the bacterial wall (endotoxins) and other components to enter the bloodstream, which may cause inflammation. Extraintestinal manifestations of ulcerative colitis may precede the diagnosis of inflammatory bowel disease, occur during remission (pyoderma gangrenosum, uveitis, spondylitis, and primary sclerosing cholangitis)

IntechOpen

The skeletal system	**Osteopenia/osteoporosis**
The liver and bile ducts	Steatosis Primary sclerosing cholangitis Autoimmune cholangitis Bile duct cancer
Joints	Arthritis of the large joints Sacroiliitis Ankylosing spondylitis
The skin	Erythema nodosum Pyoderma gangrenosum
The eye	Conjunctivitis Iritis
The vascular system	Vein thrombosis Embolism

Table 1.
Extraintestinal symptoms of ulcerative colitis.

or accompany an exacerbation (erythema nodosum, episcleritis, aphthae, and some forms of peripheral spondyloarthritis). The course of inflammatory bowel diseases in children is more severe than in adults. Extraintestinal manifestations may precede intestinal ones by months or years and may lead to false diagnoses and delayed treatment. Patients with extraintestinal manifestations often first consult other specialists, such as ophthalmologists, orthopaedic surgeons, or rheumatologists, before being diagnosed with a gastroenterological disorder. Ankylosing spondylitis or primary sclerosing cholangitis, which co-occur in patients with ulcerative colitis pose a greater health problem for some patients than the main intestinal disease(**Table 1**) [1–6].

Gastrointestinal complications are as follows:

a. Toxic megacolon (megacolon toxicum): a potentially lethal complication was observed in 3–4% of all patients with ulcerative colitis. Toxic megacolon usually occurs in patients whose whole area of the large intestine (pancolitis) has been affected shortly after the onset of the disease. Pathophysiological factors include inflammation-induced severe damage to the intestinal wall, electrolyte imbalance, and hypoproteinemia. Antidiarrheals and a barium enema may additionally contribute to the development of the complication. The removed intestine is characterised by significant thinning, fragility of the walls, and segmental mucosal atrophy. Histopathological examination shows significant hyperaemia, infiltration of all layers of the intestinal walls, and multiple small microperforations. Diagnostic criteria for megacolon toxicum involve radiological symptoms of large bowel distension, clinical symptoms (fever, HR >120/min and leukocytosis), and at least one of the following symptoms—dehydration, impaired consciousness, and decreased RR. The physical examination reveals increased tension and tenderness of the abdominal wall to palpation, as well as absent or subdued peristaltic sounds. In some cases, peritoneal symptoms occur, which may indicate an intestinal perforation. The diagnosis of toxic megacolon is based on the clinical picture and X-ray picture of the abdomen, which will show extensive distension of the colon filled with gas. A radiological criterion for megacolon is the transverse colon exceeding 6 cm in diameter in the body's midline. Laboratory tests show leukocytosis, anaemia, hypoalbuminaemia, and hypokalemia.

b. Perforation of the large intestine may further complicate toxic megacolon but it may also occur independently in a severe course of the disease. It occurs in severe, often first flares of ulcerative colitis and most often affects the left half of the colon. The clinical presentation is dominated by the symptoms of acute abdomen and peritonitis. The presence of free gas trapped within the peritoneal cavity visible in the abdominal X-ray picture or CT scan is the most reliable confirmation of the perforation.

c. Intestinal bleeding: caused by significant inflammatory lesions in the rectal and colonic mucosae. It is a life-threatening condition that can only be averted by colectomy.

d. Intestinal stricture: observed in 12% of patients with UC after 5–25 years with the condition, typically in the sigmoid colon or the rectum. However, it may occur at any time during the course of the disease. A severe course of the disease gradually leads to fibrosis and strictures in the lumen of the intestines. It is caused by the hypertrophy and thickening of the muscularis mucosa with accompanying fibrotic lesions. Their length does not usually exceed 3 cm but may reach 20–30 cm. The diagnosis of this complication based on clinical symptoms is difficult. Symptoms of strictures involve constipation, abdominal distension, sometimes more severe diarrhoea, or faecal incontinence. In the endoscopic and radiological examination, the lesions may imitate those of colorectal cancer.

e. Colorectal cancer: the most serious, if remote, consequence of ulcerative colitis is colorectal cancer. Risk factors include prolonged ulcerative colitis (over 8 years), large affected area of the large intestine, and the onset of the disease in childhood. An early diagnosis is difficult. Colonoscopy, together with multiple biopsies of all parts of the large intestine play the greatest role in diagnostics. These examinations also contribute to the detection of the characteristic precancerous lesions in the form of intestinal epithelial dysplasia. Low- or high-grade dysplasia is observed in flat, macroscopically insignificantly changed, or normal mucosa or in small irregularities or polypoid elevations in the mucosa, endoscopically detectable.

f. Perirectal lesions occur in 5–18% of patients with ulcerative colitis. They include thrombosed or prolapsed haemorrhoids, skin maceration, fissures, abscesses, and/or perianal fistulas. The majority of these lesions are secondary to diarrhoea and are characterised as acute bacterial complications. The diagnosis is based on a thorough physical examination. The main type of the internal fistula in IBD is rectovaginal fistula.

g. Gastrointestinal amyloidosis is characterised by the depositing of protein substances (amyloid) in the gastrointestinal wall leading to its thickening and disorders of the motor activity of the gastrointestinal tract [1–6] (**Table 2**).

Extraintestinal symptoms. Many patients with ulcerative colitis experience symptoms from other organs and systems. Comorbidities, also referred to as systemic complications can be divided into two groups—conditions that occur mainly in the exacerbation of colitis ulcerosa (e.g., arthritis of the large joints, iritis, and erythema nodosum) and conditions occurring independently from the activity of colitis (e.g., ankylosing and most complications from the liver and bile ducts).

Intestinal complications of ulcerative colitis	Frequency of occurence
Megacolon toxicum	3–4%
Perforation	2.5–3.5%
Haemorrhage	
Perirectal lesions • fissures • abscesses • fistulas • Haemorrhoids/prolapsed haemorrhoids	5–18%
Inflammatory polyposis	10–12%
Stricture	8–12%
Cancer	0.5–1.5%

Table 2.
Intestinal complications of ulcerative colitis.

2. Malnutrition

Malnutrition is a significant complication in children with inflammatory bowel disease that results in delayed growth and puberty. Fatigue and loss of appetite are sometimes also observed. They may imitate anorexia nervosa.

Inhibition of growth and/or puberty. The main causes include chronic inflammation, abnormal level of nutrition, and intake of glucocorticoids for medicinal purposes [2, 4, 5].

3. Hepatic lesions

Liver-related symptoms may present as hypertransaminasemia caused by the disease or as a result of the treatment (sulfasalazine, steroids, azathioprine, and parenteral nutrition). Other serious complications include autoimmune hepatitis and primary sclerosing cholangitis. Liver-related symptoms are observed in about 50% of patients with ulcerative colitis. *Primary sclerosing cholangitis* (*PSC*). A total of 90% of patients with primary sclerosing cholangitis have ulcerative colitis. Primary sclerosing cholangitis (PSC) is a chronic cholestatic liver disease of complex aetiology that leads to damage to intra- and extrahepatic bile ducts. The following factors play a part in the etiopathogenesis—genetic (HLAA1, B8, DR3), autoimmune, infectious, and environmental (the impact of diet and the gastrointestinal microbiome). The disease is characterised by the narrowing of the bile ducts that impairs the flow of the bile and leads to cholestasis. Consequently, it may result in portal hypertension, cirrhosis/liver failure, maldigestion, and malabsorption of fat and vitamins. Europe and North America report the highest incidence rate, at 4.1–16/100,000 of inhabitants. The highest incidence rate is among 20–40-year-olds. The incidence rate of PSC in the paediatric population is reported at 0.2/100,000/year, with a higher rate among the adult population, at 0.5–1/100,000/year.

The clinical manifestation is not characteristic. In 40–60%, there are no clinical symptoms, and the observed abnormal parameters of cholestasis and damage to the liver suggest primary sclerosing cholangitis.

In some patients, the skin and the sclera turn yellow, and other symptoms involve itching, fatigue, loss of body weight, weakness, epigastric pain, andor episodes of fever. PSC is a progressive condition leading to cirrhosis and liver failure. A total of 50% of patients with primary sclerosing cholangitis require a liver transplant within 10–15 years of diagnosis. A total of 50–80% of patients with PSC have a co-existing inflammatory bowel disease (ulcerative colitis more often than Lesniowski-Crohn's disease). Lesions more often affect the right colon, with the rectum remaining unaffected (free). Interestingly, only 2–4% of patients with ulcerative colitis, and 1.4–3% of those with Lesniowski-Crohn's disease have co-existing PSC. Other autoimmune conditions often co-exist in patients with PSC. They are type 1 diabetes mellitus, coeliac disease, autoimmune pancreatitis and Hashimoto thyroiditis, glomerulonephritis, and/or arthritis. *Diagnosis*. Laboratory tests reveal elevated parameters of cholestasis and damage to the liver. A total of 40–50% of patients have increased IgM and IgG, and in 20–50%, there are anti-nuclear antibodies and/or anti-smooth muscle antibodies. In 50–70% of patients, pANCA antibodies are present. Cholangio-MRI reveals the characteristic picture of strictures with subsequent dilatations of the intra- and/or extrahepatic bile ducts. Retrograde cholangiopancreatography (ERCP) is performed in the case of clinical uncertainty, or a need for treatment (sphincterotomy, stenting) and/or for cytology to confirm or exclude cholangiocarcinoma. Similarly, histopathological assessment of liver biopsies is only conducted in the case of diagnostic uncertainty. Histopathological examination reveals fibrosis around bile ducts—"onion skin" in 20–40%, inflammatory infiltrate in portal areas, the proliferation of the bile ducts, and subsequent biliary ductopenia. *Complications*. Inflammation and fibrosis lead to the development of cirrhosis of the liver. Patients with PSC are at a higher risk of developing cholangiocarcinoma and/or hepatocellular carcinoma. Primary sclerosing cholangitis is linked with an increased risk of colorectal cancer (in 9% after 10 years of diagnosis, in 31% after 20 years, and in 50% after 25 years), cholangiocarcinoma, and/or gallbladder cancer (400× greater risk). Close to 50% of gallbladder polyps in patients with PSC is malignant. 1/3 of cholangiocarcinoma in adults is diagnosed at the same time as PSC. The treatment of primary sclerosing cholangitis involves ursodeoxycholic acid, which, despite being controversial, reduces the risk of dysplasia within the large intestine. It is possible that ursodeoxycholic acid lowers the concentration of endogenic, harmful metabolites of bile acids. There has been research on the inclusion of vancomycin in the treatment of patients with PSC, but its efficacy was not proven. In the case of strictures in bile ducts and cholelithiasis, the procedure of ERCP is adopted. A liver transplant is necessary in the case of recurrent cholangitis, end-stage liver failure, portal hypertension, and/or treatment-resistant pruritus. *Autoimmune hepatitis*. In some patients, it accompanies primary sclerosing cholangitis. The clinical manifestations are not characteristic—sometimes weakness, the yellowing of the skin and the sclera, pruritis and hepatosplenomegaly. Laboratory tests reveal elevated parameters of liver damage and cholestasis, hypergammaglobulinemia, and high levels of IgG. Histopathological assessment of a liver biopsy is crucial for the final diagnosis. The treatment involves immunosuppressive drugs (glucocorticoids, azathioprine, and cyclosporine). *Cholelithiasis*. Cholelithiasis is more frequently observed in patients with Lesniowski-Crohn disease than in those with ulcerative colitis, especially with the lesions affecting the ileum terminale and after ileocecal resection (link with interrupted enterohepatic circulation). In patients with ulcerative colitis, cholelithiasis occurs noticeably and frequently following large bowel resection and is linked to the abnormal absorption and transport of bile acids. The problem may affect even 10–30% of patients. *Liver steatosis* is the most frequently observed liver pathology in the course of inflammatory bowel disease. The aetiology highlights the role of an unhealthy diet, loss of body weight, and steroid therapy. Hepatic steatosis may affect even 40% of patients with ulcerative colitis. Hepatic steatosis often correlates with the severity of the inflammatory bowel disease and often subsides once treated. *Hepatic amyloidosis*—the problem concerns 0.07% of patients with ulcerative colitis. The aggregation of amyloid in the liver leads to asymptomatic hepatomegaly. No correlation has been shown between the occurrence of amyloidosis and the advancement of intestinal lesions, the scope and duration. *Liver abscess*. It occurs more often in the course of Lesniowski-Crohn disease. Laboratory tests show leukocytosis and elevated activity of alkaline phosphatase. Liver abscesses may develop as a result of direct contact with an abdominal abscess or the hematogenous spread of inflammation. *Drug-induced hepatotoxicity*:

- 5-ASA-elevated aminotransferases
- Azathioprine/6-mercaptopurine—asymptomatic elevated aminotransferases (in 5%), vein thrombosis
- Methotrexate—steatosis, fibrosis, and cirrhosis of the liver, depending on the dose [7–16].

4. Pancreatic complications

Pancreatitis. Increased activity of amylase/lipase in the blood serum is observed in 14% of patients with inflammatory bowel disease. It is most often asymptomatic and has no link with the activity of bowel disease. *Acute pancreatitis* may be a side-effect of treatment with the following drugs—azathioprine, sulfasalazine, and mesalazine. The symptoms usually occur within the first weeks of treatment. The course of the disease is usually mild and rapidly subsides once the triggering factor has been withdrawn. Apart from the impact of the applied treatment, the pathomechanism has not been entirely determined. It may be connected with autoimmunological factors and the formation of antibodies. *Autoimmune pancreatitis*. The impact of inflammatory mediators and the presence of anti-pancreatic antibodies has been considered. It is very rarely observed in the paediatric population [1–6, 17, 18].

5. Skin lesions

Skin lesions are observed in about 3–10% of patients with ulcerative colitis. *Erythema nodosum* is an inflammatory condition that affects the subcutaneous fat in the skin and is characterised by the formation in the subcutaneous tissue of weakly delineated, flatly elevated, tender, red and warm nodules of 1–1.5 cm in diameter (the nodules may merge). They usually appear on both sides of the lower leg (less commonly on the calves), but they are not uncommon on the thighs, buttocks, arms, and torso. The nodules do not fade after 2–9 weeks, they subside without leaving scars, and they may leave post-inflammatory discolouration. It usually precedes a relapse of the intestinal condition and related gastrointestinal manifestations. However, in some patients, the course of this skin complication is independent of the activity of ulcerative colitis. It may affect even 10–15% of patients with ulcerative colitis, more of whom are women. The treatment involves the treatment of the intestinal disease, and glucocorticoids also render good results. *Pyoderma gangrenosum*. It occurs very rarely in the paediatric population with inflammatory bowel disease, affecting less than 1% of patients. Pyoderma gangrenosum most often presents in its severe, classic form (skin ulcers) or milder, pustular form. The lesions rapidly transform into ulcers affecting the skin and the superficial layer of the subcutaneous tissue. They are mainly located within the pretibial region, but they may affect every body part. They may lead to abscesses, ulcers, and osteomyelitis. Pyoderma gangrenosum does not always correlate with the activity of intestinal disease. Histopathological examination shows necrotic lesions in the skin, substantial leukocyte infiltrations, thrombosed veins, and petechiae. The healing process is difficult and leaves behind anthropic scars. The treatment involves high doses of glucocorticoids and in some cases cyclosporine and infliximab. *Sweet's syndrome* is a form of erythema exsudativum multiforme with accompanying fever and neutrophilia, also seen in patients with ulcerative colitis. Lesions may resemble erythema nodosum but steroid treatment rapidly brings improvement. *Psoriasis*. Occurs five times more frequently in patients with ulcerative colitis than in the population. It may be a side effect of the applied biological treatment. *Epidermolysis bullosa acquisita*. Following a mechanical injury, large subepithelial blisters form, often blood-filled. The lesions are most often located on the hands, the soles of the feet, in the elbow creases and behind the knees. Erosions within the oral cavity are observed in some patients. *Necrotizing vasculitis*. May lead to peripheral gangrenous lesions.

Stomatitis aphthosa occurs in around 3% of patients with ulcerative colitis. Mouth ulcers most often present as small and rather shallow erosions in the mucosal surfaces of the cheeks, soft palate, and/or the tongue. Such ulcers require differential diagnosis with moniliasis, which is another complication following severe lapses of ulcerative colitis treated with glucocorticoids and antibiotics [19, 20].

6. Rheumatoid symptoms

Arthritis may affect single or many joints, including knees, elbows, and/or hips (around 3.8%). Ankylosing spondylitis and sacroiliitis may also occur. Manifestations from the musculoskeletal system are the most common extraintestinal symptoms of inflammatory bowel disease, with as many as 25% of patients with UC affected. Arthritis may occur together with, or irrespective of the level of activity of inflammatory bowel disease. Lesions of the joints occur more often in patients with intestinal and extraintestinal complications, such as abscesses, pseudopolyps, perirectal lesions, and/or lesions in the mouth, erythema nodosum or pyoderma gangrenosum. The location of arthritis may change and may move from one joint to another. It usually lasts several weeks, rarely leading to joint deformity, and subsides following standard treatment for IBD. Patients are diagnosed with arthralgia (the presence of pain not linked with the inflammation) and spondyloarthropathies (arthritis with swelling, pain, redness, impaired mobility, and lesions seen in the imaging tests). The pathophysiology of these conditions is not fully known. *Classification*: A. Type I arthritis—type I arthropathy—axial type—typically affects several large peripheral joints (usually fewer than five), with often nonsymmetric and self-limiting lesions, and linked with the activity of the primary condition. It may precede the intestinal symptoms. It does not lead to the destruction of the affected joints. B. Type II arthritis—type II arthropathy—peripheral type—concerns at least five small peripheral joints, symmetric and with no link to the primary condition. Lesions occurring in this type are usually chronic and recurring. Synovitis occurs in both types. Synovial biopsies indicate non-characteristic lesions in the form of increased blood flow, ependymal proliferation, and mononuclear cell infiltration. Laboratory tests in arthritis are not specific. Leukocytosis, the ESR, and C-reactive protein correlate more with the activity of the intestinal disease and are of little value in the diagnostics of lesions in the joints. Synovial fluid analysis shows an increased count of leukocytes with the majority of neutrophils. Radiological analysis of peripheral joints shows mild oedema of the tissue, osteoporosis, periostitis, and exudation, usually without erosions or bode destruction. CT and/or MRI scans prove very useful for the assessment of lesions within the sacroiliac joints. Axial spondyloarthropathy is treated with relevant physiotherapy, rest, and specialist medication (sulfasalazine and mesalazine, among others)—as the only treatment of the primary condition, which, once in remission will also result in the withdrawal of the manifestations from the musculoskeletal system. Lesions in type II inflammation are often chronic and recurring, with both rheumatological and physiotherapy assistance necessary.

Ankylosing spondylitis occurs in 4–8% of patients with IDB. Men are affected more often than women. In around 60% of patients, the HLA-B27 antigen is present. The occurrence of ankylosing spondylitis is over 30 times higher in patients with ulcerative colitis compared to the general population. No correlation between the advancement of lesions in the joints and that of the lesion of the large intestine has been shown. The clinical manifestations of AS involve pain and stiffness in the lumbar spine, in particular in the morning or after a period of rest. The disease is progressing and is characterised by periods of relapse. It may lead to significant impairment of mobility. First-line treatment involves physiotherapy and in some cases immunosuppressants. *Sacroiliitis* occurs in around 14% of patients with inflammatory bowel disease but is mildly symptomatic in 90% of cases. There is no link between sacroiliitis and the activity of intestinal disease. The course is often asymptomatic, and the condition is diagnosed incidentally during radiological tests. The treatment involves sulfasalazine, analgesics, and physiotherapy. *Fibromyalgia syndrome* affects soft tissues, and its clinical manifestations are typical of the area affected. The most frequent symptoms are muscular pain and pain in the areas of tendon insertion points, for example, within the shoulder girdle, elbow joints, pelvis, knee joints, and rib attachments. In the physical examination, tenderness of the tendon insertion points is noticeable (tender points). The treatment involves anti-inflammatory and analgesic medication, as well as regular physiotherapy [1–6, 21–24].

7. Opthalmological manifestations (1%)

Ophthalmological manifestations concern mainly patients with ulcerative colitis, with the whole area of the large intestine affected and accompanying lesions in the joints. They occur in 6–60% of patients with IBD, almost twice as frequently in men as in women. These complications are typically one-sided, and their presence is linked with the activity of the primary condition. The most common ones involve watering eyes, burning eyes, pain in the eyes, light sensitivity, conjunctival hyperaemia, scleral hyperaemia, impaired visual acuity, or complete vision loss. Ophthalmological complications may also be asymptomatic. Inflammation may develop in any part of the eye. Episcleritis, together with uveitis is the most common ophthalmological complication of inflammatory bowel disease. Less frequent conditions include iritis scleritis, keratitis, and conjunctivitis. Among complications related to the treatment of IBD, cataract is often observed, which is probably linked to the prolonged use of glucocorticoids.

Iritis. It presents with blurred vision, headache and pain in the eye, photophobia, and irritated conjunctiva. *Uveitis*. Its course is often insidious and chronic. The clinical manifestations involve painful eyes, blurred vision, photophobia, and/or headaches. This disease occurs four times more frequently in women. In the physical examination, inflammatory lesions are concluded in the front area of the uvea, corneal opacity, and/or conjunctivitis. Lesions are usually both-sided. In 75% of patients arthritis also occurs. The treatment involves glucocorticoids, used topically and systemically. *Episcleritis*. Its course may be asymptomatic (2–5%) or may present as burning and sore eyes. The physical examination shows vascular injection of the ciliary body and visible inflammation in the episclera. The treatment involves treating the primary disease and topical steroids. *Cataract*. May be linked with the use of glucocorticoids.

Rare opthalmological complications are as follows:

- Central retinal vein occlusion and retinal vasculitis.
- Subepithelial keratopathy.
- Peripheral corneal ulcer and/or corneal infiltrates.
- Central serous chorioretinopathy [1–6].

8. Haematological complications

Anaemia concerns almost 30% of patients with IBD. It significantly affects the quality of life. Chronic blood loss, impaired absorption, and the impact of cytokines play an important role. Similarly, the applied treatment, involving sulfasalazine, methotrexate, and azathioprine also contributes to the condition. In the treatment of anaemia linked to ulcerative colitis, an early therapeutic intervention that is suited to the deficiencies and activity of the intestinal disease is extremely important.

Hypochromic anaemia is caused by microhaemorrhages within the gastrointestinal tract and ongoing inflammation. Anaemia caused by B12/folic acid deficiency includes autoimmune haemolytic anaemia and thrombocytopenia/thrombocytosis [1–6, 25–27].

9. Osteoporosis/osteopenia

Reduced bone mineral density has a complex mechanism and is related to deficiencies in protein and calories, abnormal absorption of calcium, vitamin D deficiency, glucocorticoid therapy, and the adverse impact of proinflammatory cytokines (TNF-alpha, IL-1alpha, IL-1Beta, and IL-6) on the bone tissue metabolism. Osteoporosis occurs in approximately 15% of patients with inflammatory bowel disease. Osteoporosis and osteopenia develop particularly often in patients with co-existing sclerosing cholangitis, probably as a result of the abnormal transportation and absorption of bile acids. It has been shown that patients with IBD statistically significantly more often experience fractures of long bones and the corpus vertebrae.

Densitometry is a screening test and should be performed in particular in groups of patients with severe IBD, especially treated with glucocorticoids [1–6].

10. Nephrological complications

In patients, especially in paediatric ones, the calcium obtained from food interacts with unabsorbed fatty acids. This leads to an increase in urine oxalate excretion, and significantly increases the risk of urolithiasis. Some studies concerning IBD mention cases of glomerulonephritis caused by concentrations of immune complexes in patients affected. Recurring urinary tract infections, hydronephrosis, and renal amyloidosis are reported relatively more frequently compared to the general population.

Urolithiasis. Occurs particularly often in patients with Lesniowski-Crohn disease and with the affected small intestine or following its resection. It develops as a result of calcium-binding with unabsorbed fatty acids.

Interstitial nephritis. Also known as tubulointerstitial nephritis is an inflammation process that develops mainly in the areas of the kidney other than the glomeruli. Those areas, that is, the renal interstitium and renal tubules become infiltrated with inflammatory cells, which leads to abnormal renal functions. The symptoms of acute interstitial nephritis may occur from the 1st day to over 2 months (on average within 3 weeks) after the triggering factor (e.g., the intake of new medication). The most common manifestations include fever and pain within the lumbar area. Chronic interstitial nephritis may be asymptomatic for many years. *Glomerulonephritis* is a group of diseases characterised by the inflammation of the glomeruli, which impairs normal kidney functions. Inflammatory cells (lymphocytes and leukocytes) and antibodies concentrate within the glomeruli that trigger the hyperplasia of the normal glomerular cells. If the inflammation is chronic, the glomeruli become fibrotic over time, and this leads to renal failure. *Infections of the urinary tract*. Frequently recurring cystitis; E.coli being the most frequently isolated pathogen. *Hydronephrosis is* caused by the obturation of the ureter by inflammatory lesions within the abdominal cavity. Renal amyloidosis [1–6, 28–30].

11. Cardiological complications

Pericarditis, including drug-induced; sulfasalazine/mesalazine [1–6, 31, 32]. Myocarditis occurs in patients with ulcerative colitis twice as frequently as in the healthy population.

12. Pulmonary complications

The following occur with a greater frequency—pulmonary vasculitis, chronic bronchitis and bronchiolitis, and bronchiectasis (more extensive and more rapidly developing compared to those of another aetiology). It is sometimes difficult to determine whether the pulmonary lesions are an extraintestinal manifestation or independent comorbidity. *Interstitial pneumonia*. Interstitial lung diseases are characterised by progressive damage to the architecture of the alveoli and the lungs, which leads to the loss of normal pulmonary functions.

Drug-induced pulmonary complications are as follows:

- Eosinophilic pneumonia/pleuritis: The clinical presentation is dominated by fever, cough, dyspnoea, and respiratory distress. The HRCT test shows ground-glass areas and the BAL fluid eosinophil greater than 25%.

- Methotrexate-related complications—after as little as 1 dose and up to 4 weeks following the last dose; folic acid does not protect from such complications. Imaging tests show diffuse lesions, interstitial infiltrates, fibrosis, and granulomas.

- Azathioprine-related complications—rarely-interstitial pneumonia; discontinuation of the medication usually leads to improvement and the withdrawal of the symptoms.

- Anti-TNFα-related complications-usually interstitial pneumonia-often in older patients, with previous lung strains and with simultaneous immunosuppressing therapy-discontinuation of treatment leads to the withdrawal of the symptoms in most patients.

Opportunistic infections. Infections with Mycobacterium tuberculosis, Pneumocystis carini, Listeria monocytogenes, Aspergillus fumigatus, Histoplasma capsulatum, and Cytomegalovirus.

The pulmonary lesions are usually either asymptomatic or oligosymptomatic. Pulmonary function tests show abnormalities in over 40% of patients. The classic thoracic X-ray in the majority of patients is non-characteristic. A High-resolution CT scan, on the other, is a helpful diagnostic tool.

Also, patients with inflammatory bowel disease develop asthma more often [1–4, 33, 34].

13. Arterial/vein thrombosis

Occurs 3–4 times more often in patients with inflammatory bowel disease compared with the healthy population. The frequency of occurrence increases with age and concerns 2–10% of patients with IBD. Vein thrombosis is the dominant condition. The treatment involves low molecular weight heparin.

Types of thrombosis are as follows:

- deep vein thrombosis.

- pulmonary embolism.

- thromboembolic lesions of intracranial vessels and/or of the eye.

The significance of these complications are mainly due to the young age of the affected patients, a large percentage of deaths and complex treatment (the use of anticoagulants in patients with gastrointestinal bleeding). It is often recurring. Vein thrombosis in the course of IBD is characterised by the atypical location of the thrombotic lesions, correlates with the activity of the intestinal disease and has a proven link with the use of glucocorticoids. Active intestinal disease with thrombocythaemia and increased activity of blood coagulation factors, as well as an increase in the concentration of homocysteine, are additional factors contributing to the development of thrombosis. Thromboprophylaxis should be adopted in patients with medium/acute exacerbation of inflammatory bowel disease [27].

14. Neurological complications

- Peripheral neuropathy
- Myelopathy
- Myasthenia

Vascular lesions in the central nervous system occur equally frequently in patients with ulcerative colitis and those with Crohn's Disease. They usually develop 5–6 years following the onset of the intestinal disease and often coincide with other extraintestinal manifestations of IBD [1–6, 35, 36].

15. Summary

- Better awareness of the initial symptoms, the course of the disease and extraintestinal manifestations, often preceding IBD may shorten the period from the onset of the symptoms to the diagnosis.
- Arthritis of the large joints, iritis, and erythema nodosum occurs mainly during the periods of the exacerbation of ulcerative colitis.
- Ankylosing spondylitis and most complications in the liver and bile ducts happen independently from the activity of the intestinal disease.
- Extraintestinal manifestations require differential diagnosis with conditions occurring independently from IBD and drug toxicity.

Author details

Sabina Wiecek
Faculty of Medical Sciences, Department of Paediatrics, Medical University of Silesia, Katowice, Poland

*Address all correspondence to: sabinawk@wp.pl

References

[1] Greuter T, Vavricka S. Extraintestinal manifestations in inflammatory bowel disease—Epidemiology, genetics, and pathogenesis. Expert Review of Gastroenterology & Hepatology. 2019;**13**(4):307-317. DOI: 10.1080/17474124.2019.1574569

[2] Konturek S. Gastroenterologia i hepatologia kliniczna. Warszawa: Wydawnictwo Lekarskie PZWL; 2006

[3] Malik T, Aurelio D. Extraintestinal manifestations of inflammatory bowel disease. In: StatPearls [Internet]. Treasure Island (FL): StatPearls Publishing; 2021

[4] Mendoza JL, Lana R, Taxonera C, et al. Extraintestinal manifestations in inflammatory bowel disease: Differences between Crohn's disease and ulcerative colitis. Medicina Clínica (Barcelona). 2005;**125**:297-300

[5] Rogler G, Singh A, Kavanaugh A, Rubin DT. Extraintestinal manifestations of inflammatory bowel disease: Current concepts, treatmrnt and implications for disease management. Gastroenterology. 2021;**161**(4):1118-1132. DOI: 10.1053/j.gastro.2021.07.042

[6] Trikudanathan G, Venkatesh PG, Navaneethan U. Diagnosis and therapeutic management of extra-intestinal manifestations of inflammatory bowel disease. Drugs. 2012;**72**:2333-2349

[7] Mertz A, Nguyen N, Katsanos K, et al. Primary sclerosing cholangitis and inflammatory bowel disease comorbidity: An update of the evidence. Annals of Gastroenterology. 2019;**32**(2):124-133

[8] Pollheimer MJ, Halilbasic E, Fickert P, et al. Pathogenesis of primary sclerosing cholangitis. Best Practice & Research. Clinical Gastroenterology. 2011;**25**(6):727-739

[9] Adike A, Carey E, Lindor K. Primary sclerosing cholangitis in children versus adults: Lessons for the clinic. Expert Review of Gastroenterology & Hepatology. 2018;**12**:1025-1032

[10] Broome U, Olsson R, Loof L, et al. Natural history and prognostic factors in 305 Swedish patients with primary sclerosing cholangitis. Gut. 1996;**38**:610-615

[11] de Vries A, Janse M, Blokzijl H, et al. Distinctive inflammatory bowel disease phenotype in primary sclerosing cholangitis. World Journal of Gastroenterology. 2015;**21**:1956-1971

[12] Deneau M, Jensen M, Holmen J, et al. Primary sclerosing cholangitis, autoimmune hepatitis, and overlap in Utah children: Epidemiology and natural history. Hepatology. 2013;**58**:1392-1400

[13] Laborda T, Jense K, et al. Treatment of primary sclerosing cholangitis in children. World Journal of Hepatology. 2019;**11**(1):19-36

[14] Deneau M, El-Matary W, Valentino P, et al. The natural history of primary sclerosing cholangitis in 781 children: A multicenter, international collaboration. Hepatology. 2017;**66**(2):518-527

[15] Fagundes E, Ferreira A, Hosken C, et al. Primary sclerosing cholangitis in children and adolescent. Arquivos de Gastroenterologia. 2017;**54**:286-290

[16] Valentino PL, Wiggins S, Harney S, et al. The natural history of primary sclerosing cholangitis in children: A large

single-center longitudinal cohort study. Journal of Pediatric Gastroenterology and Nutrition. 2016;**63**(6):603-609

[17] Lysy J, Goldin E. Pancreatitis in ulcerative colitis. Journal of Clinical Gastroenterology. 1992;**15**(4):336-339. DOI: 10.1097/00004836-199212000-00015

[18] Almeida P, Almeida C, Gompertz M, Berger Z. Association between autoimmune pancreatitis and ulcerative colitis: A report of 12 patients. Revista Española de Enfermedades Digestivas. 2020;**112**(9):682-687. DOI: 10.17235/reed.2020.6677/2019

[19] Greuter T, Navarini A, Vavricka S. Skin manifestations of inflammatory bowel disease. Clinical Reviews in Allergy and Immunology. 2017;**53**(3):413-427. DOI: 10.1007/s12016-017-8617-4

[20] Delgado T, Perez B, Laria L. Erythema nodosum: As an extraintestinal manifestation or complication in ulcerative colitis? Case reports. Inflammatory Bowel Diseases. 2020;**26**(7):e74-e75. DOI: 10.1093/ibd/izaa116

[21] Adachi Y, Hinoda Y, Takahashi H, et al. Rheumatoid arthritis associated with ulcerative colitis. Journal of Gastroenterology. 1996;**31**(4):590-595. DOI: 10.1007/BF02355063

[22] Klausen T, Amris K, Helin P. Ulcerative colitis complicating seronegative HLA-A2-B27 rheumatoid arthritis with sacroiliitis. Annals of the Rheumatic Diseases. 1992;**51**(8):1009-1011. DOI: 10.1136/ard.51.8.1009

[23] Attalia M, Singh S, Khalid R, et al. Relations between ulcerative colitis and rheumatoid arthritis: A review. Cureus. 2019;**11**(9):e5695. DOI: 10.7759/cereus.5695

[24] Engelhard S, Bajwa A, Reddy A. Causes of uveitis in children without juvenile idiopathic arthritis. Clinical Ophthalmology. 2015;**25**(9):1121-1128. DOI: 10.2147/OPTH.S83950

[25] Krzesiek E, Flis A, Iwańczak B. Frequency of anemia in ulcerative colitis in children. Polski Merkuriusz Lekarski. 2012;**33**(195):138-142

[26] Chaubal A, Pandey V, Choksi D, et al. Anemia in patients with ulcerative colitis in remission: A study from western India. Indian Journal of Gastroenterology. 2017;**36**(5):361-365. DOI: 10.1007/s12664-017-0791

[27] Jaqua N, Stratton A, Yaccobe L, et al. A review of the literature on three extraintestinal complications of ulcerative colitis: An ulcerative colitis flare complicated by Budd-Chiari syndrome, cerebral venous thrombosis and idiopathic thrombocytopenia. Acta Gastroenterologica Belgica. 2013;**76**(3):311-316

[28] Corica D, Romano C. Renal involvement in inflammatory bowel disease. Journal of Crohn's & Colitis. 2016;**10**(2):226-235. DOI: 10.1093/ecco-jcc/jjv138

[29] Ambruzs J, Larsen C. Renal manifestation of inflammatory bowel disease. Rheumatic Diseases Clinics of North America. 2018;**44**(4):699-714. DOI: 10.1016/j.rdc.2018.06.007

[30] Tokuyama H, Wakino S, Konishi K, et al. Acute interstitial nephritis associated with ulcerative colitis. Clinical and Experimental Nephrology. 2010;**14**(5):483-486. DOI: 10.1007/s10157-010-0294-

[31] Gruenhagen B, Alraies M, Vakil K, March S. Ulcerive coliced- induced miocarditis. BML Case Reports. 2014;**2014**:bcr2014204818. DOI: 10.1136/bcr-2014-204818

[32] Caio G, Lungaro L, Caputo F, et al. Recurrent myocarditis in a patient with active ulcerative colitis: A case report and review of the literaturę. BMJ Open Gastroenterology. 2021;**8**(1):e000587. DOI: 10.1136/bmjgast-2020-000587

[33] Majewski S, Piotrowski W. Pulmonary manifestations of inflammatory bowel disease. Archives of Medical Science. 2015;**11**(6):1179-1188. DOI: 10.5114/aoms.2005.56343

[34] Taveras N, Martinez A, Kumar R, et al. Pulmonary manifestations of inflammatory bowel disease. Cureus. 2021;**13**(3):e14216. DOI: 10.7759/cureus.14216

[35] Ferro J, Oliveira S, Correia L. Neurologic manifestations of inflammatory bowel diseases. Handbook of Clinical Neurology. 2014;**120**:595-605. DOI: 10.1016/B978-0-7020-4087-0.00040-1

[36] Scheid R, Teich N. Neurologic manifestations of ulcerative colitis. European Journal of Neurology. 2007;**14**(5):483-493. DOI: 10.1111/j.1468-1331.2007.01718.x

Section 3

Diagnosis of Ulcerative Colitis

Chapter 4

Histomorphological Diagnosis of Ulcerative Colitis and Associated Conditions

Jera Jeruc

Abstract

Ulcerative colitis (UC) is a chronic, idiopathic inflammatory disease that affects mainly young adults. The histologic examination of endoscopic biopsies or resection specimens plays an important part in the diagnosis and follow up of patients with inflammatory bowel disease, including UC. In this chapter, we discuss on main histological features that can be used when analyzing endoscopic biopsies, as well as features that can be evaluated in surgical samples of patients with UC. The differential diagnosis toward Crohn's disease and other mimickers is emphasized. In addition, the main complications associated with treatment and long-standing diseases, such as infection colitis and dysplasia are presented.

Keywords: ulcerative colitis, histology, biopsy, inflammatory bowel disease, inflammatory bowel disease-associated dysplasia, chronic active colitis, cryptitis, crypt abscess, CMV colitis, differential diagnosis, complications

1. Introduction

Ulcerative colitis (UC) is a chronic, idiopathic inflammatory disease that affects mainly young adults with no sex predominance. Its incidence is rising worldwide and is higher in developed countries [1–3].

The disease is characterized by relapsing and remitting mucosal inflammation, starting in the rectum and extending to proximal segments of the colon. Clinically, UC usually presents with chronic bloody diarrhea. Extraintestinal manifestations, including peripheral arthritis, primary sclerosing cholangitis, and pyoderma gangrenosum occur in about a third of patients [4, 5].

The diagnosis of UC is based on a combination of clinical presentation, endoscopic findings, histology, and the exclusion of alternative diagnoses. The histopathological examination of biopsy specimens is fundamental, not only for making a specific diagnosis but also in determining the state of disease activity and evaluating the prospect of healing and risk of relapse [6]. Even further, histology is essential in assessing the response to treatment and diagnosing complications of treatment and longstanding UC, such as dysplasia and cytomegalovirus (CMV) infection.

2. Histological characteristics of UC

For a reliable diagnosis of IBD, at least two endoscopic biopsies each should be taken from at least five sites along the ileum, colon, and rectum [7–11]. The histological features of UC include non-active inflammation, active inflammation, structural changes, and epithelial abnormalities [5, 8]. The inflammation is concentrated in the mucosa, only occasionally the inflammation may spread into the superficial part of the submucosa.

Non-active inflammation includes the presence of lymphocytes and plasma cells in the lamina propria that could be associated with edema and hyperemia. Apart from areas of ulceration, the inflammatory infiltrate in untreated UC is limited to the mucosa, diffuse or continuous without any variations in intensity or skip lesions, and its severity increases characteristically toward the rectum [5, 12, 13]. When three or more plasma cells accumulate in the mucosal lamina propria around the crypt base or between the crypt base and the muscularis mucosae, a condition is termed basal plasmacytosis [11, 14]. This phenomenon is observed already in biopsies obtained at early onset, sometimes it is the first lesion to appear. Although limited and focal in the initial phase of UC, it later spreads to more colonic segments [15, 16]. The occurrence of eosinophils in the lamina propria, between the crypts, and within the muscularis mucosae, has been associated with aggressive disease and a high risk of relapse [17].

Active inflammation is defined by the presence of neutrophils in the lamina propria, crypts, or surface epithelium. The term cryptitis is used when neutrophils are found penetrating the crypt epithelium, and crypt abscess is a term describing neutrophils occupying the crypt lumens [11]. Neutrophils infiltrating the surface epithelium lead to mucosal erosions or ulcerations, on the other hand, cryptitis and crypt abscesses are associated with crypt destruction, all features of structural changes of the mucosa [8, 18].

Structural changes of the mucosa include crypt distortion and changes in surface topography (surface irregularity). Chronic inflammation leads to irregular size and shape of crypts (e.g., branching and shortening), irregular distribution of the crypts in the lamina propria, and crypts with loss of parallelism. Crypt atrophy is defined as shortened crypts, accompanied by an increased layer of lamina propria stroma between the crypt basis and the muscularis mucosae [5, 11, 19, 20]. Irregular mucosal surface or pseudovillous transformation means wide crypt mouths giving the mucosal surface a finger-like appearance [15].

Epithelial abnormalities include surface epithelial damage, metaplastic changes, and mucin depletion. Surface epithelial damage, such as flattening, focal cell loss, erosions, and ulcers reflect the activity of the disease. Ulcers in UC colitis are always associated with mucosal inflammation in contrast with Crohn's disease, in which the surrounding mucosa can appear uninflamed [5]. In addition, UC ulcerations tend to be more superficial, broad based and continuous [21]. In severe disease, these ulcers may undermine the adjacent mucosa, finally resulting in denudation of the mucosal surface or deep penetration through the muscularis mucosae [8]. Extensive ulceration with sparing of remaining mucosal islands may give rise to inflammatory pseudopolyps, which are common in the sigmoid and descending colon, but rare in the rectum [9, 20]. Hypertrophy of the muscularis mucosae and submucosal fibrosis is rarely identified in UC [22]. Paneth cell metaplasia, a term used when pyramidal crypt epithelial cells with supranuclear eosinophilic granular cytoplasm are present in the transverse and left

DOI: http://dx.doi.org/10.5772/intechopen.102364

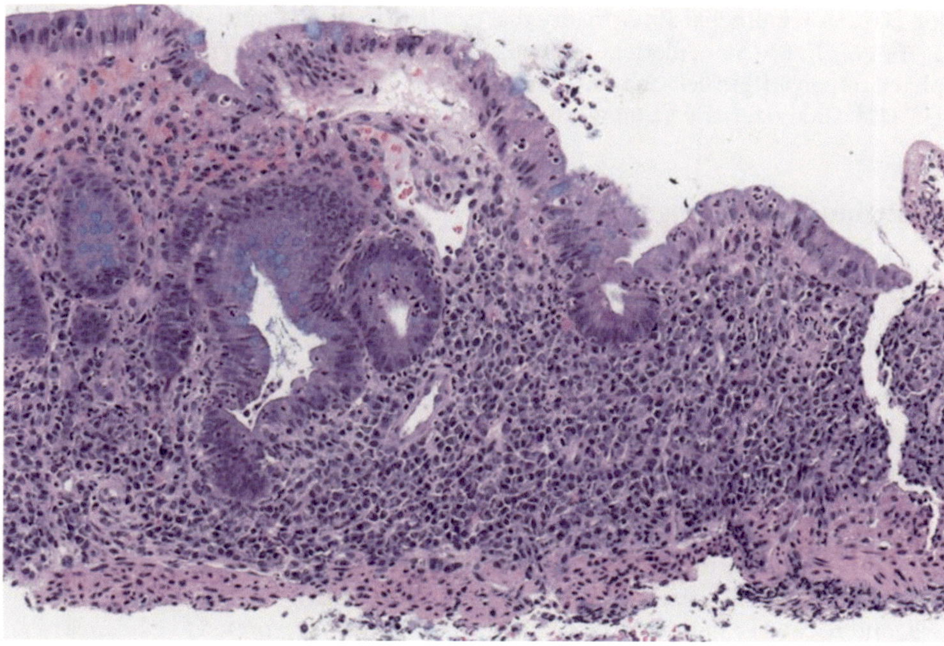

Figure 1.
Diffuse continuous inflammation with basal plasmacytosis, active inflammation with cryptitis, and structural changes including crypt distortion and atrophy. An erosion is present on the far right.

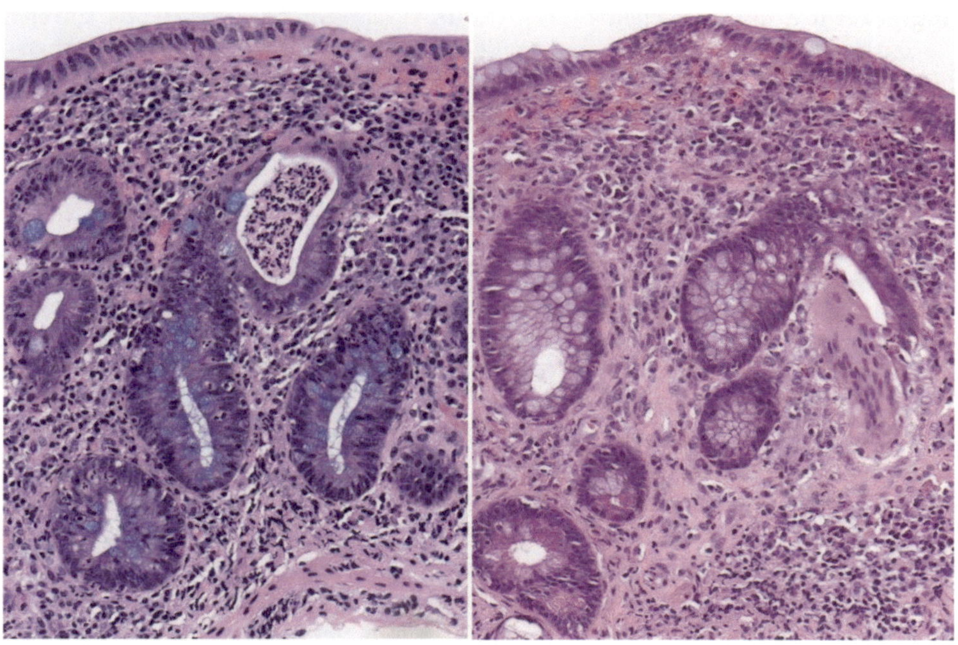

Figure 2.
Cryptitis and crypt abscess are shown on the left, while on the right Paneth cell metaplasia and cryptolytic granuloma are present.

colon [11], is an epithelial abnormality that can help in the diagnosis of long-standing UC [16, 19, 23]. Mucin depletion, defined as a reduction in number of goblet cells or depleted mucin within cells is additional epithelial abnormality frequently encountered in UC [11]. Characteristic histological features are shown in **Figures 1** and **2**.

3. Distribution of changes in UC

UC generally begins in the rectum, extending proximally in a continuous, circumferential pattern. The inflammatory infiltrate is diffuse or continuous without any variations in intensity and its severity increases characteristically toward the rectum. There are no skip-areas characteristics for Crohn's disease. The demarcation between inflamed and normal mucosa is sharp, although histological inflammation can be found in normal-appearing mucosa [22, 24]. Based on the spread of disease, three subtypes of UC are distinguished in Montréal classification—ulcerative proctitis where the proximal extent of inflammation is distal to the rectosigmoid colon, left-sided colitis, and extensive colitis when involvement extends proximal to the splenic flexure. The later also includes pancolitis [7, 25].

However, unusual inflammation patterns can occur, such as rectal sparing, cecal patch, and backwash ileitis. Rectal sparing should not be interpreted as evidence of Crohn's disease, as it can be the result of topical or systemic medications. The rectum may be spared in some adults with fulminant colitis [26, 27]. In up to 75% of patients with left-sided UC an isolated area of inflammation around the appendiceal orifice can be appreciated; this association is referred to as cecal patch [28]. In some patients with pancolitis, the ileum too is affected by acute or chronic inflammation. This condition has been termed "backwash ileitis" [29]. The ileal lesions in "backwash ileitis" are characterized by active inflammation in the villi and lamina propria, together with shortening and blunting of the villi. Focal erosions, mucous gland metaplasia, or patchy edema with mild active inflammation are features suggestive of Crohn's disease [29, 30].

4. Histological changes in different stages of the disease

UC is a chronic disease with the relapsing-remitting course and histological alterations are changing during the course of the disease. They are further influenced by medical treatment. In early-stage disease, the diagnosis of UC can be challenging due to the fact, that crypt architecture may still be preserved [17]. In longstanding disease, with widespread architectural crypt distortion and increased cellularity of the lamina propria the diagnosis of UC is more obvious. However, in this situation, rectal sparing, cecal patch, and backwash ileitis can be found that should not lead to misdiagnosis. Under treatment, the extent of involvement of the colon tends to decrease and the distribution pattern may change from diffuse (continuous) to patchy (discontinuous). Complete restoration of the rectal mucosa can be found in 34–44% of patients [5, 18]. In quiescent (clinically inactive) disease neutrophils are not observed, the mucosa may look nearly normal, however, some features, related to chronic mucosal injuries, such as architectural abnormalities, reduced crypt density, and basal plasmacytosis remain [13] (**Figure 3**). Histological mucosal healing is characterized by the resolution of crypt architectural distortion and inflammatory infiltrate. Nevertheless, the mucosa can still show some features of sustained damage, such as decreased crypt density with branching and shortening of crypts.

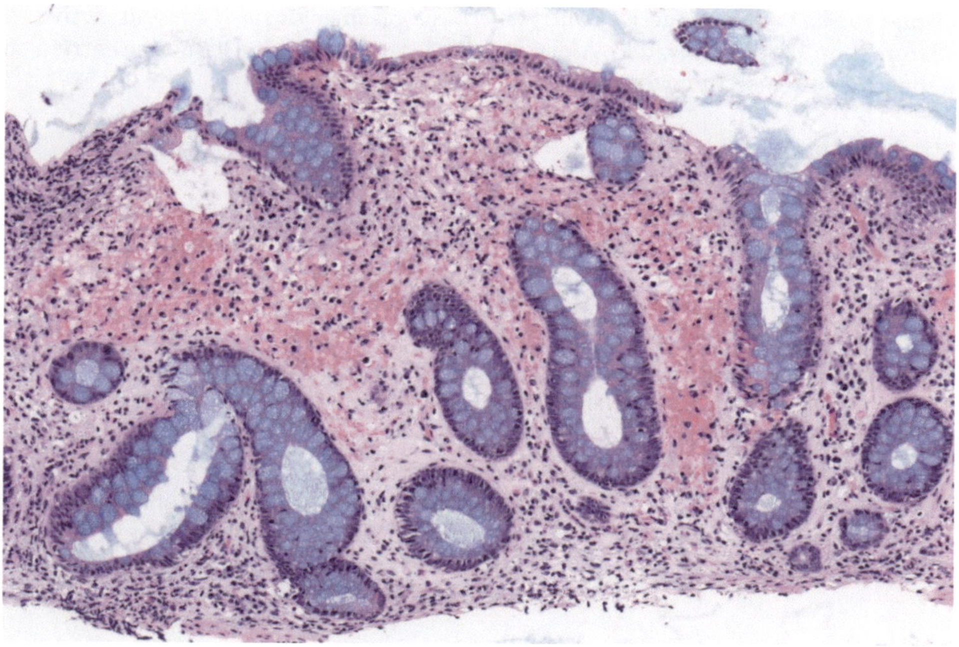

Figure 3.
Crypt architectural distortion and hypocellular stroma in quiescent disease.

5. Histologic disease activity

Assessment of disease activity is essential for developing and determining appropriate therapy in patients with UC. Disease activity and treatment response can be assessed using symptoms, biomarkers, endoscopy, and histology. Currently, clinical decision-making is predominantly based on clinical and endoscopic measures. Recently, histology has been recognized as an important prognostic factor and potential treatment target in patients with UC [31]. Both, epithelial damage in association with neutrophils and basal plasmacytosis have been proposed as markers of disease activity and the prediction of relapse. A recent meta-analysis revealed that histological remission was associated with lower rates of clinical relapse compared with those with histological activity and was a superior predictor of clinical relapse compared with endoscopic and clinical remission [32]. Furthermore, the presence of mucosal inflammation during follow-up in patients with UC was associated with a greater risk of subsequent colorectal neoplasia than in those with mucosal healing [33].

Histologically, the level of activity and the stage of the disease (e.g., flaring vs. quiescent UC) can be assessed by different scoring systems. Although more than 30 histological scoring systems in UC have been described, three have undergone extensive validation—the GS, Nancy Index, and Robarts Histopathologic Index [31, 34]. Recently a new consensus-based scoring index has been proposed, intended for both clinical practice and clinical trials that still needs to be validated [10]. Although these are not applied routinely, the pathology report should include some information on the level of activity in the biopsies to assess the effect of therapy and the risk of relapse. Pai [31] recommends that pathologists classify UC biopsies into 1 of 5 categories: normal colonic mucosa, quiescent chronic colitis without basal plasmacytosis, quiescent chronic colitis with basal plasmacytosis, chronic active colitis without basal plasmacytosis, or chronic active colitis with basal plasmacytosis. If present, active inflammation should be graded. Assessing the degree of activity should be carried out on the worst affected biopsy sample [10].

5.1 Fulminant UC

Fulminant colitis is a term used for clinically acute severe colitis, usually involving the entire large bowel, often associated with systemic illness and sometimes accompanied by colonic dilatation (toxic megacolon). It is a well-recognized mode of presentation of UC that typically requires surgical resection [35]. In fulminant UC resections show mainly acute features (**Figure 4**), while chronic changes are rarely present. With the absence of the part of classical histological changes characteristic of UC both, identification and subclassification of inflammatory bowel disease can be very difficult.

In fulminant colitis, the macroscopic appearance of the mucosa is not sufficiently distinct to differentiate UC from Crohn's disease and serositis may be observed [27, 36]. In parallel, fulminant colitis caused by UC may show Crohn's-like histological features, such as deep ulcers, transmural inflammation, and rectal sparing. There may

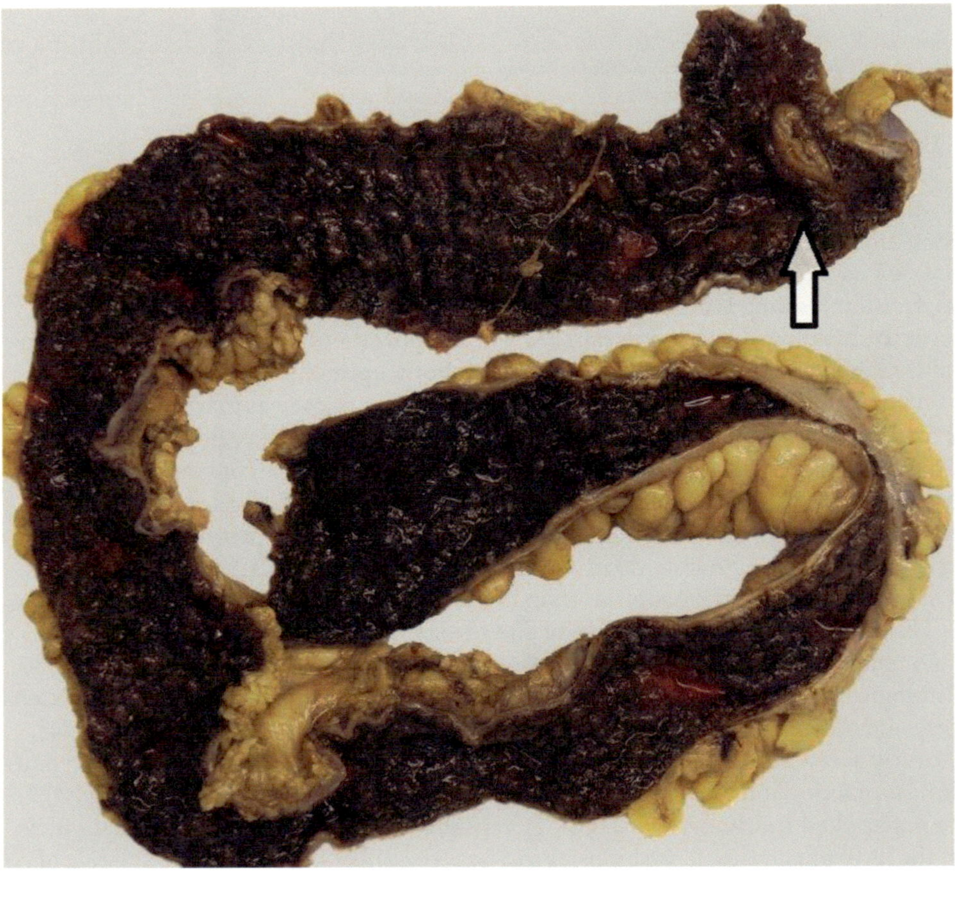

Figure 4.
Surgical resection of the colon from a patient with fulminant UC. Sharp demarcation from macroscopically normal terminal ileum is apparent (arrow).

be deep ulcerations, typically eroding down to muscularis propria in a broad-based fashion. The transmural inflammation in this setting is typically more active and diffuse, lacking discrete lymphoid aggregates. This finding does not preclude a diagnosis of UC. In a study by Swan, the two most specific predictors of a final diagnosis of Crohn's disease were granulomas and transmural lymphoid aggregates, macroscopic features were unhelpful [27]. Apparent rectal sparing is also recognized in fulminant UC, where inflammation of the transverse colon is so severe as to make the rectum look comparatively spared [37].

6. Histological mimickers of UC

The main histological feature of UC is chronic active inflammation. In addition to Crohn's disease, many conditions can mimic UC on mucosal biopsies. Besides being familiar with histological features of a wide range of diseases and conditions that can be included in the differential diagnosis, a knowledge of the clinical, endoscopic, and in some cases even imaging features is required for the pathologist to come to the right conclusion. It is, therefore, recommended that the pathologist has access to the endoscopy report and possibly also radiological and microbiological investigations [21, 22]. Some more common mimickers are addressed in the following section.

6.1 Crohn's disease

Although Crohn's and UC are frequently discussed together under the term chronic inflammatory bowel disease, distinguishing UC from Crohn's is nevertheless important. One of the reasons is that only patients with UC are considered for ileal pouch formation, because of the high risk of complications after this procedure in patients with Crohn's disease. The most common macroscopic and microscopic features distinguishing UC from colonic Crohn's disease are listed in **Table 1**. Although non-caseating epithelioid granulomas are considered a classical feature of Crohn's disease, the presence of granulomas associated with cryptolysis are now well recognized in UC and their presence should not exclude the possibility of UC [21, 38] (**Figure 2**). Rectal sparing, cecal patch, and ileal disease, all features of UC that might suggest the diagnosis of Crohn's disease were discussed in one of the previous sections. Treatment of UC can also result in patchy disease, that is, a change from continuous to discontinuous inflammation and should not lead to reclassification to Crohn's disease [26]. Transmural inflammation, another classical feature of Crohn's disease may be encountered in fulminant UC [27]. Compared to surgical resection samples, the confident distinction of UC from Crohn's disease is even more challenging in endoscopic biopsy samples where only mucosal and limited submucosal tissue is sampled. When convincing features of chronic inflammatory bowel disease are evident, but further classification is not possible, the diagnostic term inflammatory bowel disease, unclassified (IBDU) is used [5, 22].

6.2 Infective colitis

Infective colitis is one of the most important differential diagnoses of chronic inflammatory bowel disease including UC since the steroid therapy used for treating inflammatory bowel disease can have adverse results in patients with infective colitis.

Typical features	Ulcerative colitis	Crohn's disease
Localization of inflammation	Limited to the mucosa, sometimes submucosa	Transmural
Non-active inflammation	Diffuse (continuous)	Focal (discontinuous), with skip lesions
Lymphoid aggregates	Frequent in mucosa, submusosa	Common, transmural
Granulomas	Absent, except cryptolytic	Common, transmural
Active inflammation (cryptitis, crypt abscesses)	Diffuse (continuous	Focal (discontinuous)
Ulcers	Superficial	Deep, fissure-like, aphtous
Fistulae	Absent except in fulminant UC	Common
Inflammatory pseudopolyps	Common	Rare
Crypt architectural irregularity	Diffuse (continuous), marked	Focal (discontinuous)
Atrophy	Present, pronounced	Uncommon, mild
Paneth cell metaplasia	Present	Uncommon
Pyloric gland metaplasia	Rare	Present
Neuronal/muscular hypertrophy	Rare/absent	Common/present
Serositis	Absent except in fulminant UC	Present
Wall thickness	Normal	Increased
Strictures	Uncommon	Common
Fat wrapping	Absent	Common

Table 1.
Classical microscopic and macroscopic characteristics of ulcerative colitis and Crohn's disease.

One of the most common inflammatory patterns in enteric infections is the so-called nonspecific acute self-limited colitis that characteristically features intact crypt architecture with neutrophilic infiltrates of the surface epithelium. Basal plasmacytosis should not be seen as this is a marker of chronicity [39]. However, crypt abscesses and cryptitis may be present in the acute phase. As patients often do not come to endoscopy until several weeks after onset of symptoms, pathologists frequently do not see the classic histological features of acute infectious-type colitis. The protracted course of colitis, which may be seen for example in Campylobacter infections or shigellosis is more challenging to diagnose histologically as the development of "chronic" features such as crypt destruction and architectural disturbance may resemble inflammatory bowel disease including UC [40]. Extensive involvement of the surface mucosa by neutrophils is not often seen in inflammatory bowel disease and should alert the pathologist to the possibility of infection or toxin-induced injury [40]. In contrast, basal plasmacytosis, one of the earliest features of UC, crypt distortion, and irregular mucosal surface favor inflammatory bowel disease over infection [16, 19, 41]. However, in patients with early-onset UC (within 10 days of symptoms) structural changes may not yet be present [5, 42].

Lymphogranuloma venereum (LGV) and syphilis are sexually transmitted diseases caused by Chlamydia trachomatis and Treponema pallidum, respectively.

LGV and syphilitic proctitis are usually reported in men who have sex with men and can clinically mimic UC [43]. Histologically, both infections are characterized by an intense lymphohistiocytic infiltrate associated with prominent plasma cells within the mucosa and submucosa but minimal basal plasmacytosis. Characteristically, the associated acute inflammation with cryptitis and crypt abscesses is only mild to moderate. Crypt distortion and granulomas are minimal as well and Paneth cell metaplasia is rare [19, 43, 44]. Specific antibodies for T. pallidum are available that work well on paraffin-embedded tissue, however, real-time polymerase chain reaction on rectal swab specimens is the most reliable diagnostic test [43].

In addition to infections mimicking UC, in treated patients with clinical deterioration, superimposed infection, particularly CMV and Clostridium difficile should be considered [45, 46].

In some cases, diagnosis of infectious colitis is not possible on histological grounds alone. It is, therefore, vital to exclude infection by stool culture. In addition, a detailed clinical history addressing intestinal and extraintestinal symptoms, travel history, sexual history, and conditions influencing immune status should be collected [41].

6.3 Drug-induced colitis

Drug-induced colitis can show several histological patterns, one of them being a UC-like pattern with diffuse inflammation and ulceration. Histological features that favor drug-induced etiology include significant eosinophilic infiltrate, epithelial apoptosis, melanosis, cytoplasmic vacuolation, and increased intraepithelial lymphocytes [39].

Recently several monoclonal antibodies targeting immune checkpoint molecules became available for the treatment of advanced neoplasms. These immune checkpoint inhibitors (ICIs) induce immune activation and robust antitumor T-cell activity and can greatly improve survival. Following the administration of ICIs, immune-mediated adverse events including enterocolitis that can be severe are common [41, 47]. Microscopic features of ICI colitis include mixed inflammation of the lamina propria, cryptitis, crypt abscesses, crypt destruction, and granulomas [48] (**Figure 5**). In cases of distal distribution or pancolitis they may suggest UC. In ICI colitis crypt distortion, if present, is usually mild. Atrophic crypts often show marked attenuation of crypt epithelium and contain luminal apoptotic debris admixed with inflammatory cells [49]. If ICI colitis recurs, there may be chronic features such as basal lymphoplasmacytosis, crypt architectural irregularity, and Paneth cell metaplasia. Apoptosis and lymphocyte-mediated epithelial damage at the base of crypts favor ICI colitis, whereas severe inflammation, severe crypt distortion, and basal plasmacytosis favor UC [41, 50].

6.4 Segmental colitis associated with diverticulosis

Segmental colitis associated with diverticulosis (SCAD) is chronic colitis that is confined to the colonic segment containing diverticula [51]. By definition, the rectum and proximal colon are spared from inflammation [51]. SCAD is histologically characterized by a transmucosal chronic inflammation associated with crypt distortion, cryptitis, crypt abscesses, goblet cell depletion, basal plasmacytosis, or granulomas (UC-like or Crohn's disease-like pattern) [52]. However, these features are exclusively distributed in the sigmoid tract with sparing of the rectal and distal colonic mucosa [52–54]. Thus, for a correct diagnosis, it is fundamental to know the exact biopsy site

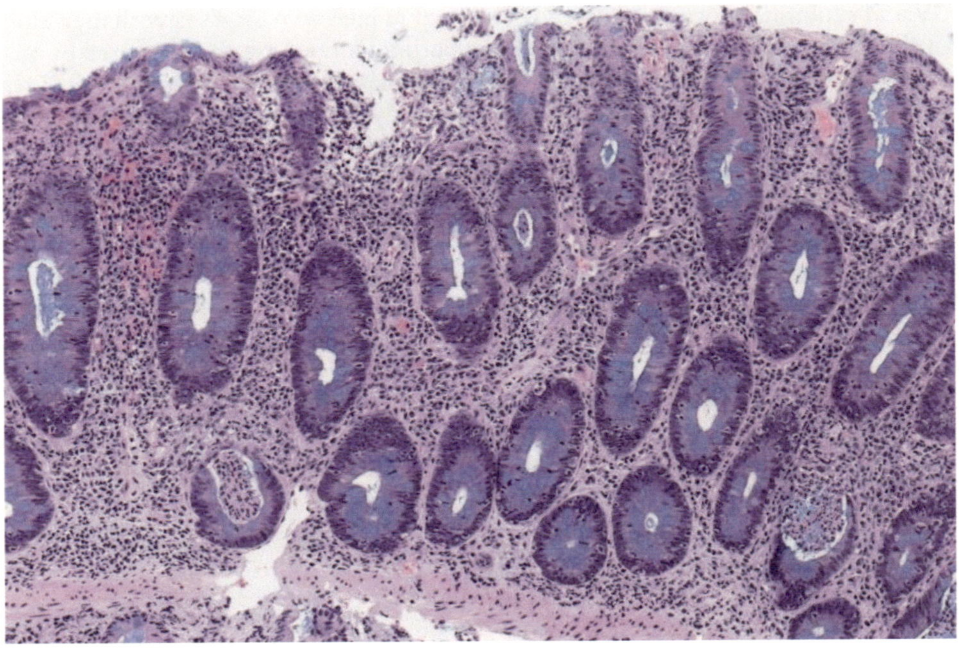

Figure 5.
Colitis associated with ICIs showing diffuse chronic inflammation with cryptitis and crypt abscesses without crypt distortion and basal plasmacytosis.

and to compare the morphology of the sigma and rectum in the differential diagnosis with IBD. In addition, patients with SCAD tend to be older compared to inflammatory bowel disease patients.

7. Associated conditions with ulcerative colitis

7.1 UC with primary sclerosing cholangitis

Primary sclerosing cholangitis (PSC) is a chronic, cholestatic liver disease, characterized by the inflammation and fibrosis of both intrahepatic and extrahepatic bile ducts, leading to the formation of multifocal bile duct strictures [55]. It is frequently associated with other diseases and a classic extraintestinal manifestation of IBD. The diagnosis of PSC may precede diagnosing the patient with IBD but can present even after colectomy in IBD patients [56]. The course of UC differs significantly when PSC is present; the most notable differences are the presence of more extensive but colitis showing lower activity. It is also more often associated with rectal sparing and so-called backwash ileitis compared with patients with UC without primary sclerosing cholangitis [56]. Another important issue is the higher incidence of carcinomas in the PSC-UC patients [56, 57].

7.2 Histological evaluation after previous surgery

Absolute indications for surgery in UC patients include uncontrolled hemorrhage, perforation, and colorectal carcinoma or dysplastic lesions not amenable to endoscopic removal. Surgery is also indicated in refractory acute severe UC or medically refractory disease [1]. The most commonly performed surgery for UC is restorative proctocolectomy with ileal pouch-anal anastomosis (IPAA) [58].

Adaptive changes of the pouch mucosa ("colonic metaplasia") are present several months after surgery in up to 87% of biopsies and consist of villous atrophy, crypt hyperplasia, and infiltration of the lamina propria by mononuclear cells, eosinophils, and histiocytes. In addition, mild ischemic changes can be observed in a few patients, while others may show features of mucosal prolapse. These changes should not be regarded as evidence of pouchitis. True pouchitis is associated with increased villous atrophy, acute and/or chronic inflammatory infiltrates, cryptitis, crypt abscesses, and ulceration [20, 59]. Based on the etiology pouchitis can be subdivided into idiopathic and secondary. Secondary pouchitis can occur in up to 30% of cases and can be classified as infectious (CMV, candida), ischemic, nonsteroidal antiinflammatory drugs-induced, collagenous, autoimmune-associated, or Crohn's disease [59]. Histology has a limited role in the evaluation of pouchitis; the main purpose for histology evaluation of the pouch is the exclusion of secondary pouchitis and dysplasia [60]. The diagnosis and differential diagnosis of pouchitis should be based on a combination of clinical, endoscopic, and histological findings [61].

When pouch biopsies show severe inflammation with neutrophils within the lamina propria and epithelium associated with erosions and ulcerations this should not lead to the reclassification into Crohn's disease. Even deep submucosal lymphoid aggregates and fistulous tracts were found in pouches excised from UC patients. A diagnosis of Crohn's disese after IPAA surgery should only be made when reexamination of the previous histological specimens shows typical pathologic features of Crohn's disese [62].

Pouchitis should be distinguished from cuffitis, which is inflammation in the columnar cuff mucosa distal to the pouch. After the IPAA procedure patients might often have residual rectal tissue, referred to as a rectal cuff, at the anastomosis between the ileum and anal canal. This area can become inflamed due to an exacerbation of UC leading to cuffitis [8, 60].

7.3 Cytomegalovirus infection and UC

In patients with UC, the risk for reactivation of latent cytomegalovirus (CMV) infection is a common complication, particularly in those with steroid-resistant disease [45]. On routine H&E stained slides, CMV typically presents as large cells, two- to four-fold larger than normal, with large amphophilic intranuclear inclusions, surrounded by a clear halo, and smaller cytoplasmic inclusions. However, CMV colitis in IBD patients tends to present with atypical, small viral inclusions, often lacking the characteristic owl-eye appearance, and it mostly affects endothelial cells in granulation tissue in ulcers [45, 63]. Therefore, CMV reactivation should be actively sought in all patients with severe colitis refractory to immunosuppressive therapy and on biopsies with prominent granulation tissue associated with large ulcers. Because the infected cells are usually scarce on limited biopsy material and morphologically less characteristic they may be missed on routine H&E stains. Immunohistochemistry, using monoclonal antibodies directed against CMV immediate early antigen, increases the diagnostic yield in comparison with H&E staining. Semiquantitative immunohistochemistry, reporting the number of infected cells and/or the number of CMV positive biopsy fragments, may have a predictive value [64].

7.4 Colitis cystica profunda

Colitis cystica profunda (CCP) is a rare benign condition characterized by cystic dilatation and misplacement of mature crypts through the muscularis mucosae into the submucosa and/or deeper layers of the bowel wall. It is a complication of various conditions including inflammatory bowel diseases, more commonly UC [65]. The condition usually affects the rectum and sigmoid colon, though it may diffusely involve the entire large bowel. It is believed to be the result of misplacement and entrapment of regenerating glands during healing. With gland formation extending deep into the bowel wall, it can be easily misdiagnosed as adenocarcinoma, particularly in endoscopic biopsies. Features favoring the diagnosis of CCP over cancer include multiple lesions, intact mucosa on the surface and no atypia on histology. Special care must be taken not to over-diagnose regenerative atypia as a well-differentiated adenocarcinoma [66].

7.5 Mucosal dysplasia and colon cancer

It has long been known that the risk of colorectal carcinoma in patients with colonic IBD is greater than in the general population [67, 68]. Recent population-based cohort studies indicate that current treatment approaches and surveillance measures have markedly reduced the risk making it more comparable to that of the general population [69]. Colorectal cancer risk, however, remains elevated in certain populations, such as those with young age at onset, long duration of disease, extensive and uncontrolled inflammation, and those with primary sclerosing cholangitis or family history of colorectal cancer [70].

Mucosal dysplasia is the best and most reliable marker of an increased risk of malignancy in patients with UC [70, 71]. Dysplasia should be distinguished into low and high degrees, using the architectural and cytological criteria of the World Health Organization [72]. In low-grade dysplasia, crypt architecture shows minimal distortion. Cytologically, the nuclei have slight hyperchromasia and the nuclear membrane has irregular edges. High-grade dysplasia is characterized by greater architectural complexity and marked nuclear pleomorphism, irregular nuclear membranes, and macronucleoli. There is more nuclear crowding and overlapping, and consequently greater nuclear stratification. Cytoarchitectural alterations not meeting the above-mentioned criteria that can also not be attributed to regeneration secondary to inflammation or medical procedure are considered "indefinite for dysplasia."

Dysplasia related to UC develops in areas with chronic inflammation and is often multifocal. Dysplasia and neoplastic lesions in UC can often be non-polypoid, flat, or ill-defined. Flat dysplasia is not endoscopically visible and can be detected microscopically in random biopsies from unremarkable mucosa. For that reason, many biopsies are performed in patients at risk to increase detection of neoplasia. The interobserver variability for dysplasia is high among pathologists, particularly for low-grade and indefinite dysplasia, making this field one of the most challenging in gastrointestinal pathology [73]. Therefore, confirmation of dysplasia by a pathologist with expertise in gastrointestinal pathology has been recommended [22]. Although discussed in past recommendations [22], recent recommendations do not encourage the use of p53 immunohistochemistry for detecting and discriminating dysplasia (**Figure 6**) [6, 8, 11].

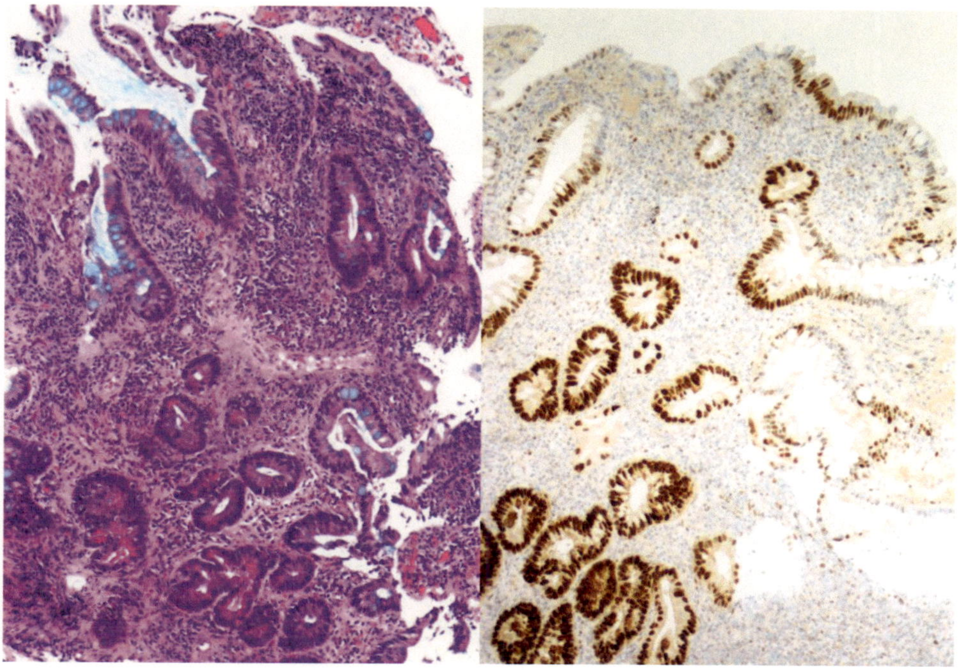

Figure 6.
Low-grade dysplasia in a patient with longstanding active UC (left) showing p53 positivity (right).

8. Conclusion

UC is a complex disease that requires a multidisciplinary approach. Histological evaluation of biopsies and resection specimens from the gastrointestinal tract plays a vital part in the management of UC patients. Despite the evolution of advanced endoscopic procedures that help in a detailed assessment of mucosa recent studies have confirmed the value of histology in predicting clinical outcomes.

Conflict of interest

The author declares no conflict of interest.

Author details

Jera Jeruc
Faculty of Medicine, Institute of Pathology, University of Ljubljana, Ljubljana, Slovenia

*Address all correspondence to: jera.jeruc@mf.uni-lj.si

References

[1] Ungaro R, Mehandru S, Allen PB, Peyrin-Biroulet L, Colombel JF. Ulcerative colitis. Lancet. 2017;**389**(10080):1756-1770

[2] Cosnes J, Gower-Rousseau C, Seksik P, Cortot A. Epidemiology and natural history of inflammatory bowel diseases. Gastroenterology. 2011;**140**(6):1785-1794

[3] Molodecky NA, Soon IS, Rabi DM, Ghali WA, Ferris M, Chernoff G, et al. Increasing incidence and prevalence of the inflammatory bowel diseases with time, based on systematic review. Gastroenterology. 2012;**142**(1):46-54

[4] Vavricka SR, Brun L, Ballabeni P, Pittet V, Prinz Vavricka BM, Zeitz J, et al. Frequency and risk factors for extraintestinal manifestations in the Swiss inflammatory bowel disease cohort. The American Journal of Gastroenterology. 2011;**106**(1):110-119

[5] Dignass A, Eliakim R, Magro F, Maaser C, Chowers Y, Geboes K, et al. Second European evidence-based consensus on the diagnosis and management of ulcerative colitis Part 1: Definitions and diagnosis. Journal of Crohn's and Colitis. 2012;**6**(10):965-990

[6] Adamina M, Feakins R, Iacucci M, Spinelli A, Cannatelli R, D'Hoore A, et al. ECCO topical review optimising reporting in surgery, endoscopy, and histopathology. Journal of Crohn's & Colitis. 2021;**15**(7):1089-1105

[7] Gajendran M, Loganathan P, Jimenez G, Catinella AP, Ng N, Umapathy C, et al. A comprehensive review and update on ulcerative colitis. Disease-a-Month. 2019;**65**(12):100851

[8] Villanacci V, Reggiani-Bonetti L, Caprioli F, Saragoni L, Salviato T, Mescoli C, et al. Histopathology of inflammatory bowel disease—Position statement of the Pathologists of the Italian Group for the Study of Inflammatory Bowel Disease (IG-IBD) and Italian Group of Gastrointestinal Pathologists (GIPAD-SIAPEC). Digestive and Liver Disease. 2020;**52**(3):262-267

[9] Magro F, Gionchetti P, Eliakim R, Ardizzone S, Armuzzi A, Barreiro-de Acosta M, et al. Third european evidence-based consensus on diagnosis and management of ulcerative colitis. Part 1: Definitions, diagnosis, extra-intestinal manifestations, pregnancy, cancer surveillance, surgery, and ileo-anal pouch disorders. Journal of Crohn's & Colitis. 2017;**11**(6):649-670

[10] Lang-Schwarz C, Agaimy A, Atreya R, Becker C, Danese S, Fléjou JF, et al. Maximizing the diagnostic information from biopsies in chronic inflammatory bowel diseases: Recommendations from the erlangen international consensus conference on inflammatory bowel diseases and presentation of the IBD-DCA score as a proposal for a new index for histologic activity assessment in ulcerative colitis and Crohn's disease. Virchows Archiv. 2021;**478**(3):581-594

[11] Magro F, Doherty G, Peyrin-Biroulet L, Svrcek M, Borralho P, Walsh A, et al. ECCO position paper: Harmonization of the approach to ulcerative colitis histopathology. Journal of Crohn's & Colitis. 2020;**14**(11):1503-1511

[12] Kleer CG, Appelman HD. Ulcerative colitis: Patterns of involvement in colorectal biopsies and changes with time. The American Journal of Surgical Pathology. 1998;**22**(8):983-989

[13] Cross SS, Harrison RF. Discriminant histological features in the diagnosis of chronic idiopathic inflammatory bowel disease: Analysis of a large dataset by a novel data visualisation technique. Journal of Clinical Pathology. 2002;**55**(1):51-57

[14] Villanacci V, Antonelli E, Reboldi G, Salemme M, Casella G, Bassotti G. Endoscopic biopsy samples of naïve "colitides" patients: Role of basal plasmacytosis. Journal of Crohn's & Colitis. 2014;**8**(11):1438-1443

[15] Schumacher G, Kollberg B, Sandstedt B. A prospective study of first attacks of inflammatory bowel disease and infectious colitis. Histologic course during the 1st year after presentation. Scandinavian Journal of Gastroenterology. 1994;**29**(4):318-332

[16] Tanaka M, Riddell RH, Saito H, Soma Y, Hidaka H, Kudo H. Morphologic criteria applicable to biopsy specimens for effective distinction of inflammatory bowel disease from other forms of colitis and of Crohn's disease from ulcerative colitis. Scandinavian Journal of Gastroenterology. 1999;**34**(1):55-67

[17] Zezos P, Patsiaoura K, Nakos A, Mpoumponaris A, Vassiliadis T, Giouleme O, et al. Severe eosinophilic infiltration in colonic biopsies predicts patients with ulcerative colitis not responding to medical therapy. Colorectal Disease. 2014;**16**(12):O420-O430

[18] DeRoche TC, Xiao SY, Liu X. Histological evaluation in ulcerative colitis. Gastroenterol Reports (Oxford). 2014;**2**(3):178-192

[19] Feakins RM. British Society of G. Inflammatory bowel disease biopsies: Updated British Society of Gastroenterology reporting guidelines. Journal of Clinical Pathology. 2013;**66**(12):1005-1026

[20] Langner C, Magro F, Driessen A, Ensari A, Mantzaris GJ, Villanacci V, et al. The histopathological approach to inflammatory bowel disease: A practice guide. Virchows Archiv. 2014;**464**(5):511-527

[21] Loughrey MB, Shepherd NA. Diagnostic dilemmas in chronic inflammatory bowel disease. Virchows Archiv. 2018;**472**(1):81-97

[22] Magro F, Langner C, Driessen A, Ensari A, Geboes K, Mantzaris GJ, et al. European consensus on the histopathology of inflammatory bowel disease. Journal of Crohn's & Colitis. 2013;7(10):827-851

[23] Tanaka M, Saito H, Kusumi T, Fukuda S, Shimoyama T, Sasaki Y, et al. Spatial distribution and histogenesis of colorectal Paneth cell metaplasia in idiopathic inflammatory bowel disease. Journal of Gastroenterology and Hepatology. 2001;**16**(12):1353-1359

[24] Annese V, Daperno M, Rutter MD, Amiot A, Bossuyt P, East J, et al. European evidence based consensus for endoscopy in inflammatory bowel disease. Journal of Crohn's & Colitis. 2013;7(12):982-1018

[25] Silverberg MS, Satsangi J, Ahmad T, Arnott ID, Bernstein CN, Brant SR, et al. Toward an integrated clinical, molecular and serological classification of inflammatory bowel disease: Report of a Working Party of the 2005 montreal world congress of gastroenterology. Canadian Journal of Gastroenterology and Hepatology. 2005;**19**(Suppl A):5a-36a

[26] Joo M, Odze RD. Rectal sparing and skip lesions in ulcerative colitis:

A comparative study of endoscopic and histologic findings in patients who underwent proctocolectomy. The American Journal of Surgical Pathology. 2010;**34**(5):689-696

[27] Swan NC, Geoghegan JG, O'Donoghue DP, Hyland JM, Sheahan K. Fulminant colitis in inflammatory bowel disease: Detailed pathologic and clinical analysis. Diseases of the Colon and Rectum. 1998;**41**(12):1511-1515

[28] Ladefoged K, Munck LK, Jorgensen F, Engel P. Skip inflammation of the appendiceal orifice: A prospective endoscopic study. Scandinavian Journal of Gastroenterology. 2005;**40**(10):1192-1196

[29] Haskell H, Andrews CW Jr, Reddy SI, Dendrinos K, Farraye FA, Stucchi AF, et al. Pathologic features and clinical significance of "backwash" ileitis in ulcerative colitis. The American Journal of Surgical Pathology. 2005;**29**(11):1472-1481

[30] Goldstein N, Dulai M. Contemporary morphologic definition of backwash ileitis in ulcerative colitis and features that distinguish it from Crohn disease. American Journal of Clinical Pathology. 2006;**126**(3):365-376

[31] Pai RK, Jairath V, Vande Casteele N, Rieder F, Parker CE, Lauwers GY. The emerging role of histologic disease activity assessment in ulcerative colitis. Gastrointestinal Endoscopy. 2018;**88**(6):887-898

[32] Park S, Abdi T, Gentry M, Laine L. Histological disease activity as a predictor of clinical relapse among patients with ulcerative colitis: Systematic review and meta-analysis. The American Journal of Gastroenterology. 2016;**111**(12):1692-1701

[33] Flores BM, O'Connor A, Moss AC. Impact of mucosal inflammation on risk of colorectal neoplasia in patients with ulcerative colitis: A systematic review and meta-analysis. Gastrointestinal Endoscopy. 2017;**86**(6):1006-1011

[34] Mosli MH, Parker CE, Nelson SA, Baker KA, MacDonald JK, Zou GY, et al. Histologic scoring indices for evaluation of disease activity in ulcerative colitis. Cochrane Database of Systematic Reviews. 2017;**5**(5):Cd011256

[35] Feakins RM. Ulcerative colitis or Crohn's disease? Pitfalls and problems. Histopathology. 2014;**64**(3):317-335

[36] Vanderheyden AD, Mitros FA. Pathologist surgeon interface in idiopathic inflammatory bowel disease. The Surgical Clinics of North America. 2007;**87**(3):763-785

[37] Haboubi N. Reporting colonic biopsies in patients with inflammatory bowel disease; a practical approach. Inflammatory Bowel Diseases. 2019;**25**(4):679-684

[38] Mahadeva U, Martin JP, Patel NK, Price AB. Granulomatous ulcerative colitis: A re-appraisal of the mucosal granuloma in the distinction of Crohn's disease from ulcerative colitis. Histopathology. 2002;**41**(1):50-55

[39] Schofield JB, Haboubi N. Histopathological mimics of inflammatory bowel disease. Inflammatory Bowel Diseases. 2020;**26**(7):994-1009

[40] Lamps LW. Infective disorders of the gastrointestinal tract. Histopathology. 2007;**50**(1):55-63

[41] Feakins R, Torres J, Borralho-Nunes P, Burisch J, Gonçalves TC, De Ridder L, et al. ECCO Topical Review on

Clinicopathological Spectrum and Differential Diagnosis of Inflammatory Bowel Disease. Journal of Crohn's and Colitis. 2021:jjab141. DOI: 10.1093/ecco-jcc/jjab141

[42] Nostrant TT, Kumar NB, Appelman HD. Histopathology differentiates acute self-limited colitis from ulcerative colitis. Gastroenterology. 1987;**92**(2):318-328

[43] Høie S, Knudsen LS, Gerstoft J. Lymphogranuloma venereum proctitis: A differential diagnose to inflammatory bowel disease. Scandinavian Journal of Gastroenterology. 2011;**46**(4):503-510

[44] Arnold CA, Limketkai BN, Illei PB, Montgomery E, Voltaggio L. Syphilitic and lymphogranuloma venereum (LGV) proctocolitis: Clues to a frequently missed diagnosis. The American Journal of Surgical Pathology. 2013;**37**(1):38-46

[45] Kambham N, Vij R, Cartwright CA, Longacre T. Cytomegalovirus infection in steroid-refractory ulcerative colitis: A case-control study. The American Journal of Surgical Pathology. 2004;**28**(3):365-373

[46] Dalal RS, Allegretti JR. Diagnosis and management of clostridioides difficile infection in patients with inflammatory bowel disease. Current Opinion in Gastroenterology. 2021;**37**(4):336-343

[47] Martins F, Sofiya L, Sykiotis GP, Lamine F, Maillard M, Fraga M, et al. Adverse effects of immune-checkpoint inhibitors: Epidemiology, management and surveillance. Nature Reviews Clinical Oncology. 2019;**16**(9):563-580

[48] Assarzadegan N, Montgomery E, Anders RA. Immune checkpoint inhibitor colitis: The flip side of the wonder drugs. Virchows Archiv. 2018;**472**(1):125-133

[49] Chen JH, Pezhouh MK, Lauwers GY, Masia R. Histopathologic features of colitis due to immunotherapy with anti-PD-1 antibodies. The American Journal of Surgical Pathology. 2017;**41**(5):643-654

[50] Adler BL, Pezhouh MK, Kim A, Luan L, Zhu Q, Gani F, et al. Histopathological and immunophenotypic features of ipilimumab-associated colitis compared to ulcerative colitis. Journal of Internal Medicine. 2018;**283**(6):568-577

[51] Lamps LW, Knapple WL. Diverticular disease-associated segmental colitis. Clinical Gastroenterology and Hepatology. 2007;**5**(1):27-31

[52] Schembri J, Bonello J, Christodoulou DK, Katsanos KH, Ellul P. Segmental colitis associated with diverticulosis: Is it the coexistence of colonic diverticulosis and inflammatory bowel disease? Annals of Gastroenterology. 2017;**30**(3):257-261

[53] Cuomo R, Barbara G, Pace F, Annese V, Bassotti G, Binda GA, et al. Italian consensus conference for colonic diverticulosis and diverticular disease. United European Gastroenterology Journal. 2014;**2**(5):413-442

[54] Tursi A, Inchingolo CD, Picchio M, Elisei W, Mangiola F, Gasbarrini G. Histopathology of segmental colitis associated with diverticulosis resembles inflammatory bowel diseases. Journal of Clinical Gastroenterology. 2015;**49**(4):350-351

[55] Chapman R, Fevery J, Kalloo A, Nagorney DM, Boberg KM, Shneider B,

et al. Diagnosis and management of primary sclerosing cholangitis. Hepatology. 2010;**51**(2):660-678

[56] Uździcki AW, Wawrzynowicz-Syczewska M. Characteristic features of ulcerative colitis with concomitant primary sclerosing cholangitis. Przeglad Gastroenterologiczny. 2021;**16**(3):184-187

[57] Krugliak Cleveland N, Rubin DT, Hart J, Weber CR, Meckel K, Tran AL, et al. Patients with ulcerative colitis and primary sclerosing cholangitis frequently have subclinical inflammation in the proximal colon. Clinical Gastroenterology and Hepatology. 2018;**16**(1):68-74

[58] Sofo L, Caprino P, Sacchetti F, Bossola M. Restorative proctocolectomy with ileal pouch-anal anastomosis for ulcerative colitis: A narrative review. World Journal of Gastrointestinal Surgery. 2016;**8**(8):556-563

[59] Zezos P, Saibil F. Inflammatory pouch disease: The spectrum of pouchitis. World Journal of Gastroenterology. 2015;**21**(29): 8739-8752

[60] Navaneethan U, Shen B. Secondary pouchitis: Those with identifiable etiopathogenetic or triggering factors. The American Journal of Gastroenterology. 2010;**105**(1):51-64

[61] Shen B, Achkar JP, Lashner BA, Ormsby AH, Remzi FH, Bevins CL, et al. Endoscopic and histologic evaluation together with symptom assessment are required to diagnose pouchitis. Gastroenterology. 2001;**121**(2):261-267

[62] Goldstein NS, Sanford WW, Bodzin JH. Crohn's-like complications in patients with ulcerative colitis after total proctocolectomy and ileal pouch-anal anastomosis. The American Journal of Surgical Pathology. 1997;**21**(11):1343-1353

[63] Zidar N, Ferkolj I, Tepeš K, Štabuc B, Kojc N, Uršič T, et al. Diagnosing cytomegalovirus in patients with inflammatory bowel disease—By immunohistochemistry or polymerase chain reaction? Virchows Archiv. 2015;**466**(5):533-539

[64] Kuwabara A, Okamoto H, Suda T, Ajioka Y, Hatakeyama K. Clinicopathologic characteristics of clinically relevant cytomegalovirus infection in inflammatory bowel disease. Journal of Gastroenterology. 2007;**42**(10):823-829

[65] Toll AD, Palazzo JP. Diffuse colitis cystica profunda in a patient with ulcerative colitis. Inflammatory Bowel Diseases. 2009;**15**(10):1454-1455

[66] Jeruc J, Drobne D, Zidar N. Diffuse colitis cystica profunda in Crohn's disease: A potential diagnostic pitfall. Journal of Crohn's & Colitis. 2019;**13**(10):1362

[67] Lashner BA. Colorectal cancer surveillance for patients with inflammatory bowel disease. Gastrointestinal Endoscopy Clinics of North America. 2002;**12**(1):135-143

[68] Bergeron V, Vienne A, Sokol H, Seksik P, Nion-Larmurier I, Ruskone-Fourmestraux A, et al. Risk factors for neoplasia in inflammatory bowel disease patients with pancolitis. The American Journal of Gastroenterology. 2010;**105**(11):2405-2411

[69] Linson EA, Hanauer SB. Epidemiology of colorectal cancer in inflammatory bowel

disease—The evolving landscape. Current Gastroenterology Reports. 2021;**23**(9):16

[70] Svrcek M, Borralho Nunes P, Villanacci V, Beaugerie L, Rogler G, De Hertogh G, et al. Clinicopathological and molecular specificities of inflammatory bowel disease-related colorectal neoplastic lesions: The Role of inflammation. Journal of Crohn's & Colitis. 2018;**12**(12):1486-1498

[71] Ullman T, Odze R, Farraye FA. Diagnosis and management of dysplasia in patients with ulcerative colitis and Crohn's disease of the colon. Inflammatory Bowel Diseases. 2009;**15**(4):630-638

[72] Nagtegaal ID, Arends MJ, Odze RD, Lam AK. Tumours of the colon and rectum. In: Lokuhetty D, White V, Watanabe R, Cree IA, editors. Digestive System Tumours. WHO Classification of Tumours. 5th ed. Lyon, France: IARC Press; 2019

[73] Odze RD, Goldblum J, Noffsinger A, Alsaigh N, Rybicki LA, Fogt F. Interobserver variability in the diagnosis of ulcerative colitis-associated dysplasia by telepathology. Modern Pathology. 2002;**15**(4):379-386

Chapter 5

The Role of the Pathologist in Ulcerative Colitis

Gayana Mahendra and Janaki Hewavisenthi

Abstract

Pathologists have an essential and wide role in the management of patients with ulcerative colitis (UC) which is a chronic inflammatory disorder of the bowel with remissions and relapses. The initial diagnosis of UC itself is challenging as the histological features vary widely with the clinical phase of the disease. Differentiating UC from other types of acute and chronic colitis, especially Crohn's disease is crucial in the management. Understanding the characteristic morphological features of UC as well as unusual morphological features of the disease are important in this task. The histological disease activity has now been identified as important in therapeutic decisions. There are several histological activity indices in UC and currently, the Nancy histological index has been recommended to be used in daily clinical practice. Identifying dysplasia associated with UC and its grading is a challenging task for the pathologist and it is a crucial step in the surveillance and management of this chronic disease.

Keywords: ulcerative colitis, histological features, diagnostic pitfalls, histological disease activity, dysplasia in ulcerative colitis

1. Introduction

Ulcerative colitis (UC) is a chronic inflammatory disorder of the colon characterized by remissions and relapses. The disease almost always begins in the rectum and extends proximally to involve the colon. In some patients, the disease is confined to the rectum (ulcerative proctitis) and in others, the inflammation extends to a variable distance along the colon in a continuous manner. The entire colon is involved in some patients (pancolitis). The clinical presentation and the disease course vary widely amongst patients. Majority of the patients present with an acute episode that clinically mimics any of the acute colitis. The patients on surveillance could show minimal clinical symptoms and minimal histological changes during the periods of remission. Some patients have continuous low activity while some may have an initial episode of active disease followed by long periods of quiescence where the accuracy of the initial diagnosis becomes questionable [1]. Some patients present with the fulminant disease either as the first attack or in an acute exacerbation and this may lead to resection of the colon as an emergency measure.

The pathologist plays a major role in the diagnosis and the management of this chronic relapsing disease. The differing clinical presentations, the chronic relapsing

IntechOpen

and remitting nature of the disease resulting in recurrent mucosal damage and healing, and the iatrogenic interventions both medical and surgical lead to a variable pathological picture (both macroscopic and microscopic) making the pathologists task a difficult one. Therefore, the diagnosis of UC should always be a combined effort of the clinician, endoscopist, and pathologist. The pathologist should be provided with information regarding clinical symptoms, their duration, the clinical course of the disease, the treatment received by the patient, and the endoscopic appearance of the bowel.

The pathologists are called upon to play various roles during the management of UC. These include the initial diagnosis of the disease and its differentiation from the other forms of colitis and in the classification of inflammatory bowel disease (IBD) in differentiating it from Crohn disease (CD). The morphological differential diagnosis of UC is wide and depends on whether the biopsies are performed during an acute relapse, in remission, or while on treatment.

Assessment of disease activity in UC is another responsibility of the pathologist. There are various clinical and endoscopic activity indices; however, histology is considered to be the gold standard in assessing the disease activity in UC [2]. There are various activity indices used by pathologists. The selection of the activity index that is used in practice is largely determined by the preference of the reporting pathologist and the responsible clinicians [3].

Pathologists are also required to identify dysplasia associated with UC. Dysplasia is an indicator of poor prognosis in UC patients, with a high risk of evolution towards invasive colorectal adenocarcinoma in the absence of treatment. Diagnosis and classification of dysplasia in UC is a challenge to the pathologist and it is a crucial step in the surveillance and management of the patients.

Basic knowledge of the histopathology of this disease is important for clinicians managing UC to interpret and act on the information provided in the pathology report. Here, the morphological features of UC are reviewed, with an emphasis on typical features as well as atypical features that could cause diagnostic pitfalls. The challenges the pathologist faces when examining the diagnostic material at different stages of the disease are highlighted. Further, the use of histological indices for the evaluation of disease activity, identification, and grading of dysplasia associated with UC are also discussed.

2. Macroscopic appearance of ulcerative colitis

UC is characterized by diffuse, continuous inflammation without skip lesions, restricted to the rectal and colonic mucosa. The bowel is characteristically filled with blood-stained dark fluid mixed with mucus. At the onset of the disease, the mucosa shows diffuse granularity, oedema, and erythema justifying the term 'red velvety' appearance. With the progression of the disease, the mucosa becomes friable with the appearance of punctate ulcers followed by irregular broad-based ulcers of various sizes. Ulceration may undermine the mucosa creating mucosal bridges. Ulcers distributed along the long axis of the colon extending down to muscularis propria are seen in UC but not the serpentine ulcers that are characteristic of CD. These mucosal changes involve the rectum and variable lengths of the proximal colon in continuity. The distal colon is more severely diseased than the proximal colon. The margin between the inflamed and normal mucosa is distinct and abrupt.

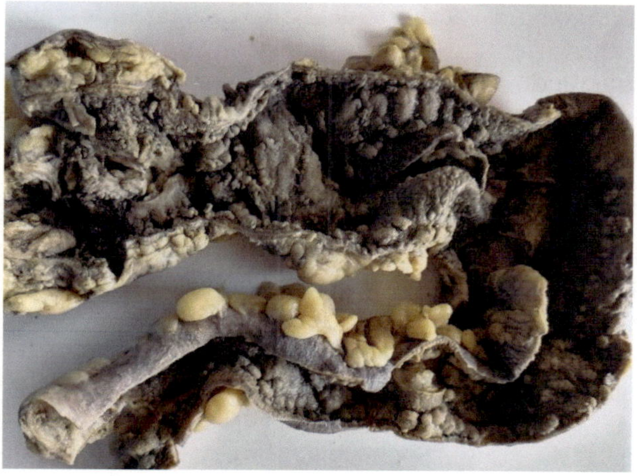

Figure 1.
Macroscopic appearance of the colon in UC showing involvement of the entire colon with ulceration and pseudopolyp formation.

Against a backdrop of mucosal ulceration, there are islands of non-ulcerated residual and regenerating mucosa, bulging into the lumen creating inflammatory pseudopolyps which are usually small, multiple, and bizarre in shape. Sometimes these pseudopolyps could be large and may mimic malignancy (**Figure 1**) [4].

The mucosa is atrophic and smooth with the absence of mucosal folds in long-standing UC. In the quiescent stage of UC, the mucosa may appear normal or exhibit diffuse granularity and inflammatory pseudopolyps.

The extent of UC is classified according to the Montreal classification as follows [5];

a. Ulcerative proctitis	Only the rectum is affected
b. Left-sided or distal UC	Colonic involvement distal to the splenic flexure
c. Extensive UC or pancolitis	Involvement of the colon extending proximal to the splenic flexure

3. Microscopy appearance of ulcerative colitis

For the optimum assessment of the microscopy, the pathologist should be supplied with adequate and good-quality colonoscopic biopsies. The endoscopist should obtain samples from the ileum, at least four colonic sites, and the rectum, with a minimum of two biopsies from each site [6].

Biopsies from each colonic segment should be submitted in separate containers for each colonic segment, which should be accurately labeled. This is of paramount importance as the pathologist has no means of identifying the separate colonic segments/sites based on histology. This in turn will hinder the pathologists' attempts at mapping the pattern and distribution of disease activity throughout the colon.

Samples should be fixed immediately by immersion in buffered formalin solution before transport and should be accompanied by clinical information, including endoscopic findings, duration of disease, and current treatment. It is important to sample both endoscopically normal as well as abnormal mucosa as there could be histological activity identified in even endoscopically normal mucosa [7, 8]. Proper orientation of the biopsy during tissue embedding is important as tangentially sectioned biopsies hinder the assessment of the crypt architecture. Serial sectioning is also vital as certain focal features like granulomas may appear at different levels. However, the ideal number of sections is not defined and varies with the laboratory. At least two tissue levels, and preferably three, are advisable [2]. Some laboratories produce step-sections on two slides, but this may incur extra costs. Routine staining with hematoxylin and eosin is appropriate. Special stains and immunohistochemistry are not routinely necessary for the diagnosis or classification of IBD [2].

3.1 Main histological characteristics of ulcerative colitis

The knowledge of the normal histology of the gastrointestinal mucosa is essential for the optimal interpretation of biopsy specimens in IBD. Four main histological characteristics are assessed in the diagnostic process of IBD.

3.1.1 Crypt architectural abnormalities

Normal colonic crypts are straight, parallel, and extend from the surface, up to the muscularis mucosae. The crypt architecture is assessed based on the crypt size, crypt branching, crypt shortening, and variability in inter-crypt spacing. The crypt architectural distortion observed in UC is characterized by irregularly arranged, dilated, branched, fused, and shortened crypts. The crypt size and spacing could vary. This is a manifestation of ongoing inflammation and regeneration [9]. However, the crypts in the anorectal junction and ileocaecal junction can show minor abnormalities resembling architectural distortion due to regional variations. Another point to remember is that the crypt architecture should not be assessed close to lymphoid aggregates as these could result in distortion.

3.1.2 Cellularity in the lamina propria

Lymphocytes and plasma cells are always found in the colorectal lamina propria (LP). Normally, these chronic inflammatory cells are most dense in the upper third of the mucosa and their density decreases towards the base, resulting in the 'plasma cell gradient'. The absence of the plasma cell gradient is accepted as normal in the caecum and ascending colon. The cellularity in the LP varies depending on the anatomical site of the colon. In general, the caecum and the right colon are most cellular with a progressive decrease in the cellularity from the right to the left side. Dense lymphoid tissue may be found in the normal large bowel, particularly in the rectum. The abundance of eosinophil granulocytes varies a lot between normal individuals and is found to have a seasonal and geographic variation and is more in the right colon and the ileum than the left colon [2, 10].

Abnormal cellularity of the LP refers both to increased and altered distribution of cell types that are normally present. Basal plasmacytosis or plasma cells extending below crypt endings in more than two foci in a biopsy is considered to denote an increase in chronic inflammation (**Figure 2**).

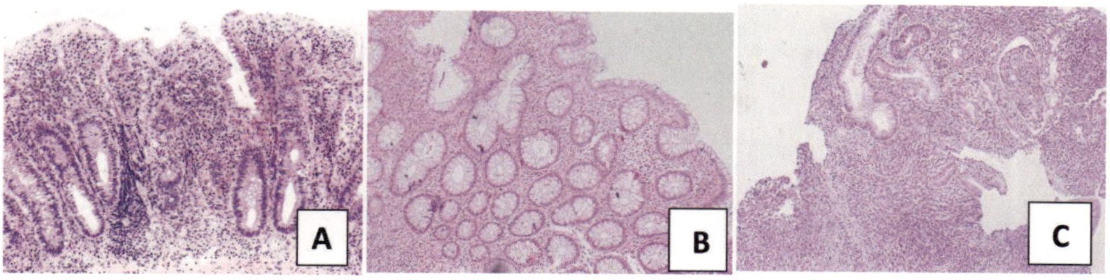

Figure 2.
Main histological features of UC. (A) Basal plasmacytosis and mucin depletion. (B) Villiform surface, variation in size and shape and branching of crypts. (C) Surface ulceration, diffuse heavy inflammatory cell infiltrate in the lamina propria and crypt abscess formation ((A–C): H&E ×200).

3.1.3 Neutrophil granulocytes in the lamina propria

Normal colonic mucosa does not contain neutrophils except a few scattered neutrophils, that may occur as a result of bowel preparation [11]. Neutrophils are the hallmark of activity in IBD/UC. These are found in the LP or they can infiltrate the crypt surface epithelium (termed cryptitis) or enter the lumen of crypts forming crypt abscesses (**Figure 2**).

3.1.4 Epithelial abnormalities

These include mucin depletion, surface epithelial damage, and metaplastic changes. Mucin depletion can be defined as a decreased number of goblet cells or decreased amount of intracellular mucin. Focal epithelial cell loss, flattening, erosions, and ulcers denote epithelial damage and reflect the activity of the disease. Metaplastic changes are seen in the form of Paneth cell or pyloric gland metaplasia. None of these findings is disease-specific and might be observed in UC, CD, and other types of colitis.

Working definitions of some of the microscopic features of IBD/UC are given in **Table 1** [11].

3.2 Typical histological features of ulcerative colitis

The histologic findings in UC vary depending on the clinical phase of the disease and the grade of inflammatory activity. The histological features that define chronicity are crypt architectural distortion, crypt atrophy, diffuse mixed lamina propria inflammation, basal plasmacytosis, basally located lymphoid aggregates, and Paneth cell metaplasia [9]. Inflammatory activity is defined by the presence of neutrophils. Neutrophilic cryptitis, crypt abscesses, hemorrhage, erosions, ulceration, and necrosis are features of active inflammation.

It is convenient to divide the histologic appearances into those seen inactive disease, resolving disease, and disease in remission.

3.2.1 Active ulcerative colitis

The characteristic features of acute UC include architectural distortion which is more in the distal colon than the proximal bowel, diffuse chronic inflammatory cell infiltrates

Microscopic abnormality	Definition	Additional remarks
Crypt distortion	Branching, loss of parallelism, irregularity, tortuosity, dilatation, and variation in shape and size of the crypts	Should not be assessed adjacent to crypt abscesses/lymphoid aggregates/follicles Anal transition zone/columnar cuff unsuitable for assessment
Crypt branching	Two or more branched crypts in a well-oriented biopsy	Branching between mucosal hillocks is normal
Crypt atrophy	Crypt shortening, with an increased gap between crypt base and muscularis mucosae Additional evidence is the wider spacing of crypts; >1 crypt diameter between crypts (normal: 6 crypts/mm in a biopsy with muscularis mucosa)	Caution adjacent to lymphoid aggregates/follicles Anal transition zone/columnar cuff is unsuitable for assessment Mucosal oedema may mimic atrophy
Villiform/irregular mucosal surface	Undulating or broadly villiform surface Wide crypt mouths	
Basal plasmacytosis	Plasma cells at the base of mucosa. May separate crypts from muscularis mucosae but not always sub cryptal Loss of plasma cell gradient	Basal plasma cells are normal in the caecum and the ascending colon
Basal lymphoid aggregates	Nodular collections of lymphocytes with or without germinal centres. It may be seen between muscularis mucosae and crypts	One or two transmucosal lymphoid nodules can be seen in normal mucosa; can extend across muscularis mucosae. Pathological aggregate may be difficult to distinguish from normal
Cryptitis	Neutrophils in the crypt epithelium	
Crypt abscess	Neutrophils in crypt lumen	Often located near the crypt base
Granuloma	A discrete collection of at least five epithelioid macrophages	Consider crypt rupture as a cause. Serial sections may help
Mucin depletion	Unequivocal reduction of goblet cell mucin in the crypt epithelium	Mucin in normal mucosa may be reduced near lymphoid follicles. Depletion can reflect bowel preparation
Ulceration/erosion	Loss of epithelium replaced by 'immature' granulation tissue or the presence of a fibrinopurulent exudate An ulcer extends more deeply than the muscularis mucosae while an erosion does not	It May be difficult to differentiate ulcer and erosion The epithelium can denude artifactually during biopsy procedures or processing
Paneth cell metaplasia	Pyramidal crypt epithelial cells with supranuclear eosinophilic granular cytoplasm	Normal in the caecum and right colon, probably as far as the splenic flexure
Diffuse chronic inflammation	An overall increase in chronic inflammatory cell density throughout the biopsy/biopsies	The caecum and ascending colon may have a higher density of chronic inflammatory cells
Patchy chronic inflammation	Areas of increased chronic inflammatory cell density in a background of variable cellularity	

Microscopic abnormality	Definition	Additional remarks
Focal chronic inflammation	Well circumscribed foci of increased chronic inflammatory cell density in a normocellular background	Differentiate from lymphoid aggregates
Focal active inflammation	Focal crypt infiltration by neutrophils in the absence of significant inflammation in the adjacent LP	Uncommon in UC but could be seen in early or treated UC

Table 1.
Working definitions of histological features seen in UC/IBD.

extending up to the muscularis mucosae, and neutrophil infiltration. The neutrophils seem to migrate directly from capillaries into the crypt epithelium (cryptitis) and often form crypt abscesses. Ulcers covered with granulation tissue and regenerative epithelium could be seen. The surface epithelium may take an undulating or low villiform appearance. The inflammation may extend into the superficial submucosa but the muscularis propria and serosa remain free of inflammation, except in fulminant colitis.

Neutrophils are predominant within the lumina of the crypts in UC and comparatively small numbers are seen migrating between the epithelial cells. Crypt abscesses are the precursors of mucosal ulceration and inflammatory polyp formation. In severe active UC, crypt abscesses burst into the loose submucosal tissues and there is a tendency to spread beneath the mucosal membrane, which sloughs off leaving an ulcer. The remaining mucosa is relatively raised from the ulcerated area and forms 'inflammatory pseudopolyps'.

The inflammatory damage to the crypts produces a variety of degenerative and regenerative changes in the crypt epithelium. There is loss of mucin from goblet cells, often with enlargement and hyperchromatism of nuclei of the absorptive cells. Such changes must not be mistaken for dysplasia. In the presence of attenuated or restituting superficial epithelium, the changes in the crypts are almost certainly reactive [1].

There is a heavy diffuse infiltrate of inflammatory cells in the LP. These include neutrophils, lymphocytes, plasma cells, eosinophils, and mast cells. The presence of deep plasma cells is characteristic of longstanding UC. Many eosinophils may be seen in the LP in some of the biopsies but the role of eosinophils in UC is uncertain and has been subject to many studies [10]. Lymphoid aggregates, that may show germinal centres, are common in UC. These are situated basally between crypt bases and the muscularis mucosae (**Figure 3**). Epithelioid granulomas, which are a hallmark of CD, are not identified in UC, where only foreign body granulomas evolved as a response to mucin from ruptured crypts (termed cryptolytic granulomas) are observed.

3.2.2 Resolving ulcerative colitis

With the resolution of disease, the numbers of inflammatory cells of all types show a variable density, therefore, the LP could be either hyper or hypocellular. Further, the distribution of inflammatory cells becomes uneven. The goblet cell population returns to normal. The crypt architecture will show variable evidence of distortion, depending on the severity of the attack. The crypts may appear short and branched, the changes invariably being more marked distally. The resolution may occur at different rates in different parts of the colon, and this may give rise to the false impression of segmental disease (**Figure 4**).

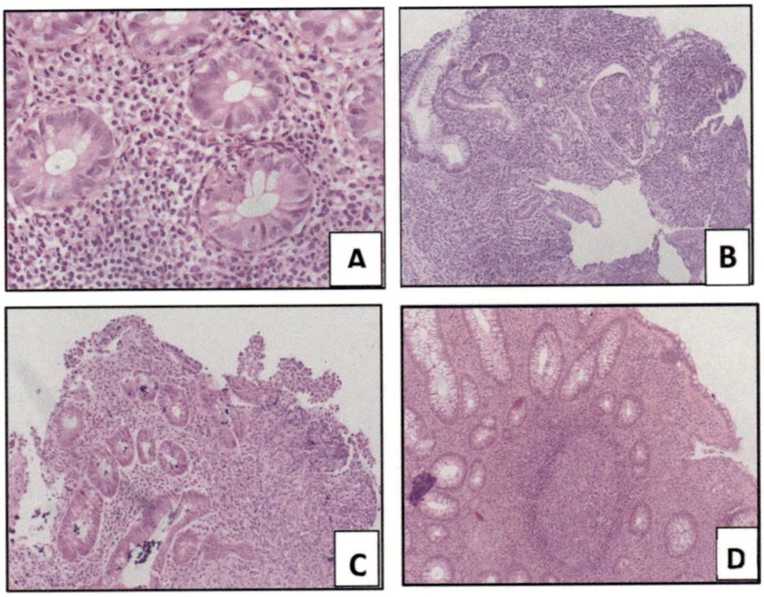

Figure 3.
Histological appearances of active UC. (A) Depletion of mucin in the epithelium, cryptitis, heavy infiltrate of lymphocytes, plasma cells, and eosinophils in the LP (H&E ×400). (B) Marked crypt distortion and crypt abscess formation. (C) Surface ulceration. (D) A lymphoid aggregate with the germinal centre formation in the LP ((B–D): H&E ×200).

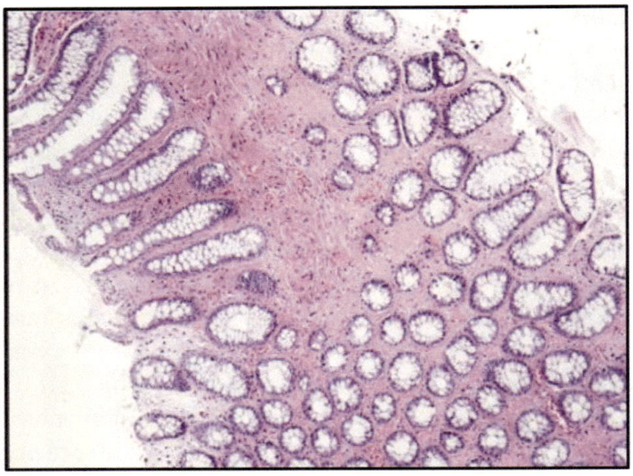

Figure 4.
Resolving UC; a mild crypt architectural distortion, normal mucin content in the glands, hypocellular LP, no activity (H&E ×100).

3.2.3 Quiescent ulcerative colitis

Varying degrees of crypt atrophy and distortion are the hallmarks of the quiescent disease. Active inflammation is absent. The muscularis mucosa is thickened and a characteristic finding in UC, especially in rectal biopsies, is the double muscularis mucosae [1]. Paneth cell metaplasia in the left colon and pyloric-type metaplasia in any location of the colon are also features of chronic disease [1].

Although most UC patients have some residual changes of previous damage, such as crypt distortion, atrophy, and Paneth cell metaplasia, it has become increasingly recognized that a group of UC patients may show complete resolution with no evidence of previous disease [12, 13]. This must always raise the question of whether the original diagnosis is UC or infective colitis. In such situations, a careful review of the previous clinical records including the initial biopsies and ancillary investigations may be of help [1].

4. Unusual morphological patterns of ulcerative colitis

There are some exceptions to the classic morphological patterns described above, that may lead to diagnostic confusion. A summary of the unusual morphologic patterns of disease in UC is noted in **Table 2**. Pathologists need to recognize these patterns to avoid falling into a diagnostic trap.

4.1 Morphological features of treated ulcerative colitis

Endoscopically or histologically discontinuous disease may be observed in the setting of medically treated UC. This occurs as a result of uneven healing [6]. The same process may also lead to absolute or relative rectal sparing in 30–40% of patients [9]. As patchiness of the disease and rectal sparing mimicking CD is commonly seen in treated UC, evaluation of disease distribution to subtype IBD should not be attempted in this setting. This emphasizes the importance of pre-treatment histology and the value of communication between the clinician and the pathologist.

4.2 Appendiceal 'skip' lesions and the 'caecal patch' in ulcerative colitis

Appendiceal involvement is demonstrated in about 75% of the total colectomies performed for UC. This may be continuous with extensive colitis or may represent a 'skip lesion' of UC with involvement of the more distal colon only [9]. Such a skip lesion may raise the suspicion of CD and be erroneously considered as a contraindication for pouch surgery. The mucosal inflammation in the appendix may extend to the appendiceal orifice and contiguous large bowel as a periappendiceal patch.

Similar to the appendiceal skip lesion, there could be isolated involvement of the caecum and/or ascending colon, which is discontinuous with the left-sided colitis. It is shown that patchy right-sided inflammation in patients with left-sided colitis has

1. Treatment effect
2. Appendiceal 'skip' lesion and 'caecal patch'
3. Ileal involvement
4. Rectal sparing
5. Paediatric UC-initial presentation
6. Fulminant colitis

Table 2.
Unusual patterns of disease in UC.

little clinical significance but should be recognized by pathologists to prevent a false diagnosis of CD in this setting [14].

It is also interesting that in appendices removed for possible acute appendicitis, inflammation confined to the mucosa with associated crypt distortion should raise the possibility of an appendiceal involvement in UC.

4.3 Involvement of the ileum

Ileitis is found in about 10% of patients with UC, the extent of involvement varying from 50–250 mm [1]. The mucosal changes are similar to those seen in the colon and are always in continuity with the disease in the large bowel. The involvement of the ileum is associated with an open dilated and incompetent ileocaecal valve. Although the term 'backwash ileitis' is in common use for this condition, it is not necessarily accurate as evidence for such a mechanism is not yet proven [1]. This condition should not be confused with CD of the terminal ileum which typically shows longer lengths of involvement and is normally associated with chronic active inflammation, and other features of CD. Unfortunately, strict histopathologic criteria for backwash ileitis have not been defined [15].

4.4 Rectal sparing

According to traditional belief, UC is a diffuse continuous disease that begins in the rectum and extends proximally, without skip areas. The term 'absolute rectal sparing' refers to the rectum with a normal endoscopic appearance and normal histology. Another term sometimes used is 'relative rectal sparing', in which the rectum has inflammation that is less severe than the more proximal colon [16]. Rectal sparing and patchiness of inflammation are seen in medically treated UC, especially with therapeutic steroid enemas. This too emphasizes the importance of the provision of clinical details to the pathologist. The pathologists should also be vigilant not to interpret these findings as definite evidence of CD.

4.5 Ulcerative colitis in pediatric populations

Pediatric-onset of IBD can show fewer characteristic symptoms and histological findings than adult-onset IBD. In general, diagnostic biopsies from children with UC often show less severe inflammation, fewer architectural abnormalities, and less epithelial injury despite extensive disease [2, 6, 17, 18].

The available evidence strongly suggests that UC in children is typically a pancolitis with variable degrees of inflammation on histology [16]. In a subset of pediatric patients, relative rectal sparing and patchy inflammation both endoscopically and histologically may occur at the pre-treatment stage of UC. These features are also observed in treated pediatric patients presumably similar to adults. In a minority, absolute rectal sparing occurs [16]. It is prudent not to preclude the diagnosis of UC in children when these atypical features are present. The precise reason why pre-treatment stage pediatric patients have a higher prevalence of rectal sparing compared to adults is unclear. Younger age (<10 years) at presentation and shorter duration between the symptoms and endoscopy are proposed explanations [19].

4.6 Fulminant ulcerative colitis

Fulminant colitis is defined as severe, acute inflammation of the colon with associated systemic toxicity. Most cases (89%) of fulminant colitis represent IBD, with the remainder relating to ischemia or infection, amongst other aetiologies [20].

In fulminant UC, the inflammatory cell infiltrate extends beyond the mucosa with thinning of the wall. There is separation and oedema of the muscle layer known as myocytolysis. There is diffuse haemorrhagic necrosis of the mucosa, deep fissuring ulcers, and transmural polymorphous inflammation. Unlike in classical UC where the serosa is shiny and intact, there is a purulent or seropurulent exudate seen on the peritoneal surface in many cases of fulminant colitis. The bowel wall is also markedly thinned out and dilated and this usually occurs in the region of the transverse colon. Macroscopic features, such as dilation, skip lesions, rectal sparing, linear ulcers, terminal ileal disease, pseudopolyps, and creeping fat, are poor discriminators of UC and CD, in the setting of fulminant colitis.

5. Histological differential diagnosis of ulcerative colitis and diagnostic pitfalls

5.1 Infective colitis

Infective colitis may clinically mimic acute UC. However, most cases of infectious colitis demonstrate a histological pattern of acute colitis, which may be diffuse, patchy, or focal, without evidence of architectural distortion. Less commonly, chronic infectious colitis may produce a histological pattern of chronic active colitis resembling IBD. Most of these cases have no specific diagnostic features on histological examination and in such cases, knowledge of the clinical history and correlation with serologic studies or stool cultures are required for diagnosis.

Some features help in differentiating acute self-limiting colitis from UC in the acute stage. In acute self-limiting colitis, the neutrophils are plentiful in the LP and are more superficially arranged. In UC, the neutrophils are predominant within the lumina of the crypts and comparatively small numbers are seen migrating between the epithelial cells [1]. Chronic changes, such as crypt distortion in UC, take about 4–6 weeks to develop and this could, therefore, cause a diagnostic difficulty in the early stages of the disease.

In amoebic colitis, presenting as chronic active colitis, there could be trophozoites of *Entamoeba histolytica* in biopsy material and identifying the trophozoites becomes crucial because, if immunosuppressive therapy is started for presumed IBD in these patients, it can result in perforation due to fulminant amoebic colitis. Superimposed infection with many organisms can occur with established UC and cytomegalovirus (CMV), campylobacter and *Clostridium difficile* are some of the important secondary infections to be considered when UC presents with an acute exacerbation [21].

5.2 Chronic ischaemic colitis

Chronic ischemia may produce a pattern of chronic active colitis and can present a difficult differential diagnosis. Chronic or recurrent ischemia may cause significant crypt distortion, Paneth cell metaplasia, and chronic active inflammation, all features which mimic UC. However, atrophic and regenerative changes in the epithelium, hyalinization of the LP, and the presence of microthrombi in the adjacent mucosa should suggest ischemia [21]. Overall, in ischemia, the chronic active inflammation is mild relative to the degree of epithelial injury [21]. Further confounding this differential diagnosis, UC has been reported to cause a hypercoagulable state, particularly in genetically predisposed patients. In this setting, a superimposed arterial and venous thrombosis may occur, leading to severe steroid-refractory colitis [21].

5.3 Diverticular disease-associated colitis (DAC)

Chronic active colitis resembling UC may be seen in the setting of diverticulosis. In addition, diverticulosis is a relatively common disease of the elderly and, thus, both diverticulosis and IBD (either CD or UC) may coexist in the same patient. Unlike chronic active colitis of UC, DAC is confined to segments involved by diverticular disease, most commonly the sigmoid colon, and, by definition, spares the rectum. However, UC and diverticular colitis may in some cases represent overlapping entities, as a small subset of diverticular colitis patients has progressed to typical rectosigmoid UC and DAC may respond to medical therapy utilized for IBD [21].

5.4 Drug-induced colitis

Some forms of medication-induced colitis may demonstrate chronic active colitis, which may enter the differential diagnosis of UC. Nonsteroidal anti-inflammatory drugs (NSAIDs) may result in the reactivation of UC. However, in some patients, this group of drugs has also been implicated in initiating UC [1].

The most useful histological feature in distinguishing NSAID-related colitis from UC is an increase in apoptotic bodies in the crypt epithelium and lymphocytes and mononuclear cells of the superficial LP. The morphological changes that occur with NSAIDs include a generalized increase in chronic inflammatory cells in the LP, a prominent eosinophil infiltrate, increased intra-epithelial T lymphocytes and thickening of the subepithelial collagen plate may resemble eosinophilic colitis, lymphocytic colitis, and collagenous colitis, respectively [1].

5.5 Diversion colitis

Diversion colitis develops in segments of the bowel that have been excluded from the fecal stream, such as in a Hartmann's pouch. This chronic inflammatory condition usually develops within a few months to several years following surgical diversion, and typically regresses completely within 3–6 months of re-establishment of the fecal stream [22]. The disease may mimic IBD on biopsy samples and may show crypt atrophy, distortion, and lymphoid hyperplasia, involving the mucosa and/or submucosa. Symptomatic patients can show superimposed cryptitis, crypt abscesses, and superficial aphthous-type erosions or frank ulceration.

This warrants the importance of obtaining a biopsy of the segment at the time of the surgery to get a baseline analysis and review of the clinical, radiological, and endoscopic information prior to diagnosis.

5.6 Crohn disease (CD)

In most instances, UC and CD may be readily distinguished from each other pathologically, particularly when each exhibits classic histological features assisted by clinical data and other ancillary investigations. There are several circumstances in which the 'classic' morphological features that help to distinguish UC from CD are altered or absent. When these atypical morphological features are present, they may mimic CD (**Tables 3** and **4**). Most of these atypical features have already been discussed in Section 3.

5.6.1 Granulomas in UC

Approximately 30–40% of CD cases contain either mucosal or mural, non-necrotic granulomas [22]. When present, it is a helpful feature to confidently diagnose CD, especially in mucosal biopsies. Granulomas in CD are composed of loose collections of CD 68 immunostain positive epithelioid histiocytes. When there is rupture of a crypt or extravasated mucin in UC, there could be the formation of a granuloma which is termed a 'cryptolytic granuloma' that could be difficult to

Pathological feature	Ulcerative colitis	Crohn's disease
Disease distribution	Diffuse and continuous	Segmental
Rectal involvement	Almost always (adults)	Occasionally
Disease severity	Increased distally	Patchy and variable
Ileal involvement	Occasional ('backwash')	Often
Inflammation of the colonic wall	Superficial (mucosal)	Transmural
Transmural lymphoid aggregates	Rare, underneath ulcers	Any location
Fissures	Rare superficial in fulminant colitis	Deep, any location
Sinuses and fistulas	Absent	Present
Granulomas	Related to ruptured crypts 'cryptolytic granuloma'	Not crypt-related and are epithelioid cell granulomas

Table 3.
Classic morphological features helpful in differentiating UC from CD [13].

1.	Discontinuous or patchy disease ('caecal patch')
2.	Absolute or relative rectal sparing
3.	Inflammatory changes in the ileum ('backwash' ileitis)
4.	Treatment-related change
5.	Granuloma formation
6.	Transmural inflammation

Table 4.
Unusual morphological patterns of UC that may mimic CD.

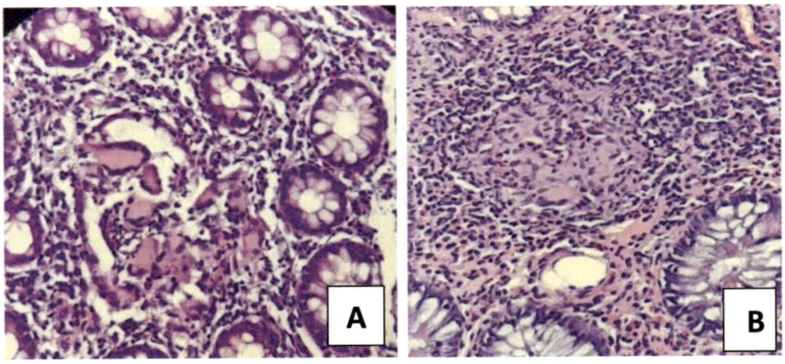

Figure 5.
(A) Cryptolytic granuloma following a rupture of a crypt in UC. Extravasated mucin, multinucleated giant cells, and inflammatory cells are seen. (B) Epithelioid cell granuloma formed by histiocytic cells in CD ((A and B) H&E ×400).

distinguish from granulomas of CD (**Figure 5**). Examination of multiple tissue levels that will demonstrate the relationship between granulomas and the crypt epithelium is a helpful measure in this situation. Cryptolytic granulomas often contain an admixture of neutrophils and lymphocytes, in addition to foamy macrophages and multinucleated foreign body-type giant cells and these are not usually seen in CD-related granulomas [22].

5.6.2 Transmural inflammation in UC

In CD, transmural lymphoid aggregates are seen randomly in the wall of the bowel. In fulminant UC when superficial fissuring ulcers that extend into the deep submucosa or superficial muscularis propria are present and in toxic megacolon when myocyte necrosis and serosal inflammation are prominent, there could be mural mononuclear inflammation. However, in contrast to CD, these do not form typical discrete lymphoid aggregates and are usually seen underlying the areas of severe ulceration [22]. Thus, lymphoid aggregates in areas under intact mucosa are not a feature of UC and, in fact, favor a diagnosis of CD.

5.6.3 CD with UC-like features

Typical features of CD such as granulomas, fissuring ulcers, and transmural lymphoid aggregates are seen less commonly in the colon compared to the small intestine [15]. Therefore, some cases of colonic CD may mimic UC by demonstrating only superficial mucosal involvement without inflammatory changes in the submucosa or muscularis propria, diffuse and continuous disease, and even pancolitis. Nearly 20% of CD patients develop colitis without the involvement of the upper GI tract [22]. In these cases, careful evaluation of colonic and ileal biopsies for granulomas, identifying focal or patchy inflammation and activity within the LP, identifying transmural lymphoid aggregates in resections, correlation with a detailed clinical history and imaging will be of help in differentiating UC from CD.

6. Indeterminate colitis (IC) and inflammatory bowel disease unclassified (IBDU)

In up to 5% of IBD cases, an exact classification of IBD into UC or CD proves difficult due to either the overlapping histological features of the two diseases or to the fact that UC and CD represent two ends of the spectrum of a single disease [1, 6].

Several different terms have been used to refer to this condition, including 'indeterminate colitis' (IC), 'inflammatory bowel disease unclassified' (IBDU), 'chronic inflammatory bowel disease unclassified', and 'chronic idiopathic inflammatory bowel disease not otherwise specified'. The European Crohn's and Colitis Organization (ECCO) and the European Society of Pathology (ESP) jointly addressed the ambiguous usage of this terminology, in their consensus report in 2013 [6]. Accordingly, the term IBDU could be used for patients with chronic colitis who have IBD based on the clinical history, but endoscopy and histology of the biopsies show no definitive features of either UC or CD [6]. This term is reserved for biopsy examination as the post-operative examination of resections of such IBDU cases usually provides definitive evidence of UC or CD.

The entity of IBDU is more common in the pediatric population. The possible reasons for this being more colitis than ileitis occurs in CD in early cases and the presence of rectal sparing in UC in the pediatric population [6]. Upper GI biopsies are particularly helpful in these cases.

The pathological diagnosis of IC is made only on resected specimens with the presence of overlapping features or the absence of a clear diagnostic pattern to distinguish CD from UC.

Usually, macroscopically IC shows diffuse disease with involvement of transverse and right colon and less severe inflammation in the distal colon. There is extensive ulceration. Microscopy confirms extensive ulceration with a sharp transition to normal adjacent mucosa and multiple V-shaped ulcers lacking surrounding inflammation. The overlapping histological features of IC are given in **Table 5**.

It makes no difference whether the large bowel resection is called 'UC' or 'IC', but CD needs to be excluded conclusively since an ileal pouch-anal anastomosis (IPAA)/'pouch' procedure is generally contradicted in CD.

• Severe mucosal and wall involvement
• Non-aggregated transmural inflammation
• Fissures reaching the muscularis propria
• Discontinuous pattern
• Diffuse mucosal disease with normal ileum
• Deep mural lymphoid aggregation
• Non-necrotizing granulomas in lymph nodes
• Anal fistula

Table 5.
Overlapping histological features in indeterminate colitis (IC).

7. Measuring the disease activity in ulcerative colitis

The complete assessment of disease activity in UC involves symptomatic evaluation, physical examination, measurement of laboratory indices, endoscopic visualization, and the histological assessment of the mucosal inflammation [3]. However, measuring disease activity using all these different parameters is cumbersome and time-consuming in practice and will delay therapy. In routine clinical practice, the disease activity and subsequent medical treatment are usually assessed largely by the clinical symptomatology. Histological assessment of the degree of inflammation is the gold standard for evaluating the true disease activity but its conventional use is limited owing to its inconvenience, invasiveness, and cost [3].

Traditionally, clinical and endoscopic remission were the two main therapeutic targets for UC. However, up to 40% of patients in clinical and endoscopic remission show persistent histological activity [2]. Furthermore, histological activity predicts the worst outcome and histological inflammation represents a significant risk factor for the subsequent development of UC-related colorectal neoplasia. Therefore, histological remission is now increasingly regarded as an important therapeutic target for UC [2].

There are about 30 histological activity indices in IBD, that have been introduced over the last few decades [23]. These systems use different stepwise grading scales for the assessment of inflammation which is used as the basis of grading the disease activity. These scales have four to seven steps and quantitatively assess the following features—architectural changes in the mucosa, chronic inflammatory cell infiltrate, amount and location of neutrophils within the mucosa, crypt abscess formation, erosion, and ulcers.

Of these scores, the 'Geboes score' developed in 2000 has been the most widely used and can serve as an independent risk factor for disease progression in UC [24, 25]. The more recent 'Nancy histological index' (NHI) and 'Robarts histopathological index' (RHI) both from 2016 have proven feasible, easy to use, and are the most extensively validated [26, 27]. There is currently no general agreement on which index should be used. The 2020 ECCO position paper concluded that the NHI can be recommended for daily clinical practice and for clinical trials both the NHI and RHI are feasible [2].

RHI requires assessment of four features which include ulceration/erosion, neutrophils in the epithelium, neutrophils in the LP, and the chronic inflammatory cell infiltrate. Each of the features is subdivided on a scale of 0–3 to calculate the ultimate disease activity score. This may reduce its clinical usefulness and probably is more useful for clinical trials and in research. In NHI, three main histological characteristics which include ulceration, the acute inflammatory cell infiltrate and the chronic inflammatory cell infiltrate are assessed. The NHI is defined by a 5-level classification ranging from grade-0 (absence of significant histological disease activity) to grade-4 (severely active disease) (**Table 6**) [27].

In the NHI, chronic inflammation includes lymphocytes, plasma cells, and eosinophils and it is assessed without quantification. Furthermore, if neutrophilic inflammation is present, regardless of extent, the degree of chronic inflammation is not assessed.

It has been shown that both NHI and RHI have a similar degree of inter and intra-observer agreement and share equivalent feasibility in terms of time taken for scoring the biopsies [28].

Histological criteria and defining features	Disease activity	Score
Ulceration Loss of colonic crypts replaced with immature granulation tissue or presence of a fibrinopurulent exudate	**Severe**	4
Acute inflammatory cells infiltrate Presence of neutrophils in LP and/or epithelial cells	**Moderate to severe** Presence of multiple clusters of neutrophils in LP and/or in the epithelium that is easily apparent.	3
	Mild Few or rare neutrophils in LP or in the epithelium that are difficult to see	2
	Absence Assess the chronic inflammatory cell infiltrate	
Chronic inflammatory infiltrate Presence of lymphocytes and/or plasma cells and/or eosinophils in LP	**Moderate to severe** Presence of an increase in chronic inflammatory cell number that is easily apparent	1
	Mild No or mild increase in chronic inflammatory cell number	0

Table 6.
Nancy histological index (NHI).

Despite the development and validation of novel histologic scoring systems, there are no agreed definitions for histologic healing and remission. Histologic healing is the ultimate goal of the treatment and could be defined as complete normalization of the mucosa [7]. What constitutes complete normalization needs to be precisely defined. Rare architecturally distorted crypts should not be overinterpreted as evidence of persistent architectural abnormalities. A rare, branched crypt can be seen even in a normal colon. Furthermore, the crypts in a normal rectum often do not extend to the muscularis mucosae [7].

The best definition of histologic remission in UC is also unclear. Traditionally, this has been regarded as persistent architectural abnormalities without neutrophilic (active) inflammation, with varying degrees of lymphoplasmacytic inflammation. The presence of mucosal eosinophils is allowed [7]. Ideally, remission includes clinical, endoscopic, and histological resolution, which is called complete remission.

8. Dysplasia andv malignancy in ulcerative colitis

The risk of colorectal carcinoma (CRC) is increased in patients with long-term UC compared to the general population. Carcinogenesis in UC is inflammation-driven and has a different pathway than usual colorectal carcinogenesis. Epithelial cells acquire early mutations of TP53 and KRAS genes and no mutations of APC genes, while in non-inflammatory carcinogenesis of the colon, APC mutation is the earliest event [7].

Epithelial dysplasia is the precursor lesion of UC-associated CRC. The features associated with increased risk of dysplasia/CRC in UC include the duration of the disease, the anatomical extent of the disease, early age of onset, concomitant sclerosing cholangitis, family history of CRC, and endoscopic/histological activity of the disease [29]. The prognosis of CRC in IBD may be worse than CRC in the general population and shows higher mortality [9].

8.1 Colorectal dysplasia in ulcerative colitis

The presence of dysplasia in endoscopic biopsies is the most reliable marker of cancer risk. There are no specific clinical features related to dysplasia in UC. Most cases of dysplasia occur in the left/distal colon, and this mirrors the higher incidence of UC-associated colorectal carcinoma (CRC) in the rectosigmoid region. The endoscopic appearance of dysplasia is categorized according to the SCENIC classification and includes visible and invisible lesions. The visible lesions are subdivided into polypoidal (either pedunculated or sessile) and non-polypoidal (superficial, flat, depressed [29].

Dysplasia of the colorectum is defined as an unequivocal epithelial alteration that remains confined within the basement membrane within which it originated. The microscopic features of dysplasia in UC are based on a combination of cytoarchitectural features of the crypt epithelium that remains confined to the mucosa and are identical to those used in the general assessment of dysplasia elsewhere [9]. Dysplasia is classified according to either the Riddell or the Vienna system [30, 31]. In the Riddell system, there are four categories for dysplasia, which are negative, indefinite, low grade, and high grade. The Vienna system has five categories with the addition of invasive carcinoma.

The most common histological subtypes of dysplasia include intestinal (adenomatous) and serrated types [29]. Regardless of these subtypes, dysplasia is divided into low grade and high grade according to the cytoarchitectural features. In low-grade dysplasia (LGD) the crypts may be tubular and/or villous or serrated and they show either no or only mild crypt budding or crowding. The dysplastic cells show enlarged, hyperchromatic nuclei with a high nuclear/cytoplasmic ratio, nuclear stratification limited to the basal half of the cytoplasm, and clumped chromatin or multiple small nucleoli. In serrated dysplasia, the dysplastic cells may show hypereosinophilic, mucin depleted cytoplasm, or a microvesicular epithelium that is similar to the sporadic sessile serrated adenomas. These atypical nuclear features usually involve both the crypt and surface epithelium.

High-grade dysplasia (HGD) exhibits enlarged nuclei with marked nuclear hyperchromasia, pleomorphism, stratification involving the full thickness of the cytoplasm, increased mitoses, and loss of nuclear polarity. It shows complex glandular architecture with crowding, cribriforming, complex branching, and budding [29].

The category indefinite for dysplasia refers to ambiguous epithelial alterations that cannot with certainty be classified either as negative or positive for dysplasia. Some of the settings in which indefinite for dysplasia is considered are shown in **Table** 7.

8.2 Some issues in histopathological reporting in UC-associated dysplasia

A. Examination of multiple biopsies is necessary to rule out the possibility of dysplasia confidently, as dysplasia is also identified in endoscopically normal mucosa.

B. The active and resolving phase of UC may cause diagnostic difficulties as the damaged or the regenerative epithelium may harbor mucin depleted cells and

1.	Atypical cytological features in an inflammatory background where differentiating regenerative change from LGD/HGD could be difficult
2.	Marked cytological atypia in the crypt bases where surface maturation cannot be assessed due to ulceration or poor orientation
3.	Various artifactual cytological changes occur as a result of poor histological techniques—processing, cutting, staining
4.	Only a very small focus (only a few crypts) shows dysplasia.

Table 7.
Some settings where indefinite for dysplasia are considered.

atypical nuclear changes, such as enlargement, hyperchromasia, stratification, and brisk mitoses. Careful observation for surface maturation, which is a feature in reactive conditions helps to solve this problem. Another good practice is to perform colonoscopic surveillance during a period of remission of UC.

C. Inter-observer agreement amongst pathologists for dysplasia associated with UC is suboptimal. Poor reproducibility is seen mainly in indefinite dysplasia and LGD groups. (6). Reporting the biopsies for dysplasia ideally by two histopathologists will help to overcome this problem. A review of the biopsies with the diagnosis of dysplasia by a more experienced gastrointestinal pathologist, before any surgical intervention is undertaken, will optimize the management of these patients.

D. Adenomas can arise in both affected and non-affected mucosa in UC patients. They are treated like any other adenomas by complete local excision. The stalk or the tissue around the base of the lesion needs to be examined carefully to confirm that these are adenomas or part of a more widespread area of dysplasia associated with UC.

E. Colonic biopsies of patients treated with immunosuppressive agents, such as cyclosporin for severe UC, are known to show 'pseudo dysplastic' changes in the

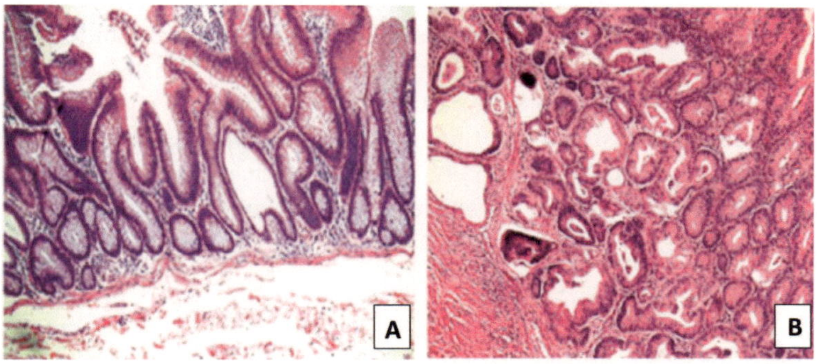

Figure 6.
Dysplasia in UC. (A) Flat low-grade dysplasia with villous configuration. There is no significant pleomorphism or loss of polarity (H&E ×100). (B) High-grade dysplasia with crowding glandular proliferation (H&E ×100). Reprinted by ([21], pp. 178-192). Published by Oxford University press and digestive science publishing Co Limited.

epithelium [32]. Perhaps the most helpful feature is that the 'pseudo-dysplasia' induced by cyclosporin is strikingly diffuse, with many, and sometimes all, crypts showing similar changes, a pattern not usually seen in UC associated dysplasia. Therefore, the clinician needs to alert the pathologist to the fact that the patient has been on cyclosporin and that the pathologist in turn should be cautious when diagnosis dysplasia in this situation (**Figure 6**).

8.3 The demise of the term 'DALM' in ulcerative colitis

A diagnosis of dysplasia is made on biopsy material taken from a polyp or a mass evident on endoscopy was historically termed 'dysplasia associated lesion or mass' (DALM) and was considered as an indication for colectomy to rule out the possibility of invasive malignancy. In 2015 SCENIC international consensus statement on the surveillance and management of dysplasia in IBD, abandoned the term DALM and replaced it with endoscopically visible and non-visible lesions [33]. With advancements in endoscopic polypectomy and endoscopic mucosal resections (EMR), the concept of DALM is now outdated because most lesions that are noninvasive can be removed using these techniques [1].

8.4 Carcinoma in ulcerative colitis

Carcinomas arising in UC are mostly similar to their counterpart in non-colitis patients except for the background colitis. However, there are some features that are more frequent in UC-associated carcinomas. The tumors could be multiple and often are flat lesions with ill-defined edges, therefore, these tumors are easily felt than seen. Histologically there is a higher incidence of high-grade tumors and mucinous subtypes [1].

9. Conclusions

The pathologist plays a vital role in the diagnosis and follows up of patients with UC. The histological features in the biopsies vary widely depending on the stage of this chronic relapsing and remitting disease, making the differential diagnosis lengthy and challenging. The final diagnosis should be ideally concluded at a clinico-pathological meeting. Understanding the typical and atypical histological features of UC is vital in the task of differentiating UC from other types of colitis, mainly CD. Histological disease activity and identifying histological remission are increasingly considered important therapeutic targets. Identifying dysplasia associated with UC and its grading is a crucial step in the surveillance and management of this chronic disease.

Acknowledgements

The authors gratefully thank Dr. D.T.T. Jayasinghe and Dr. R.D.K. Medonza, Postgraduate trainee in Histopathology, Faculty of Medicine, University of Kelaniya, for their assistance in photomicrography.

Author details

Gayana Mahendra* and Janaki Hewavisenthi
Faculty of Medicine, Department of Pathology, University of Kelaniya, Sri Lanka

*Address all correspondence to: baggmahendra@yahoo.co.uk

References

[1] Jain D, Warren BF, Riddell RH. Inflammatory disorders of the large intestine. In: Shepherd NA, Warren BF, Williams GT, Greenson JK, Lauwers GY, Novelli MR, editors. Morson and Dawson's Gastrointestinal Pathology. 5th ed. Chichester, West Sussex, UK: Wiley-Blackwell; 2013. pp. 552-635

[2] Magro F, Doherty G, Peyrin-Biroulet L, Svrcek M, Borralho P, Walsh A, et al. ECCO position paper: Harmonization of the approach to ulcerative colitis histopathology. Journal of Crohn's and Colitis. 2020;**14**. DOI: 10.1093/ecco-jcc/jjaa110

[3] Mahendra BAGG, de S. Hewavisenthi SJ. The role of the pathologist in the assessment of disease activity in ulcerative colitis. Journal of Diagnostic Pathology. 2018;**13**. DOI: 10.4038/jdp.v13i1.7749

[4] Chen W-C, Lashner B, Wang M-H. Giant inflammatory pseudopolyposis mimicking colonic tumor in an ulcerative colitis patient. American Journal of Gastroenterology. 2016;**111**. DOI: 10.14309/00000434-201610001-01738

[5] Satsangi J, Silverberg MS, Vermeire S, Colombel JF. The Montreal classification of inflammatory bowel disease: Controversies, consensus, and implications. Gut. 2006;**55**:749-753. DOI: 10.1136/gut.2005.082909

[6] Magro F, Langner C, Driessen A, Ensari A, Geboes K, Mantzaris GJ, et al. European consensus on the histopathology of inflammatory bowel disease. Journal of Crohn's and Colitis. 2013;**7**:827-851. DOI: 10.1016/j.crohns.2013.06.001

[7] Pai RK, Jairath V. vande Casteele N, Rieder F, Parker CE, Lauwers GY. The emerging role of histologic disease activity assessment in ulcerative colitis. Gastrointestinal Endoscopy. 2018;**88**:887-898. DOI: 10.1016/j.gie.2018.08.018

[8] Mahendra BAGG. Is endoscopic examination alone adequate in determining the extent of disease in ulcerative colitis? The Srilanka Journal of Surgery. 2006;**24**:18-21

[9] Kellermann L, Riis LB. A close view on histopathological changes in inflammatory bowel disease, a narrative review. Digestive Medicine Research. 2021;**4**. DOI: 10.21037/dmr-21-1

[10] Loktionov A. Eosinophils in the gastrointestinal tract and their role in the pathogenesis of major colorectal disorders. World Journal of Gastroenterology. 2019;**25**:3503-3526. DOI: 10.3748/wjg.v25.i27.3503

[11] Feakins RM. Inflammatory bowel disease biopsies: Updated British Society of Gastroenterology reporting guidelines. Journal of Clinical Pathology. 2013;**66**:1005-1026. DOI: 10.1136/jclinpath-2013-201885

[12] Kleer CG, Appelman HD. Ulcerative Colitis: Patterns of involvement in colorectal biopsies and changes with time. American Journal of Surgical Pathology. 1998;**22**: 983-989. DOI: 10.1097/00000478-199808000-00008

[13] Levine TS, Tzardi M, Mitchell S, Sowter C, Price AB. Diagnostic difficulty arising from rectal recovery in ulcerative colitis. Journal of Clinical Pathology. 1996;**49**:319-323. DOI: 10.1136/jcp.49.4.319

[14] Mutinga ML, Odze RD, Wang HH, Hornick JL, Farraye FA. The clinical

significance of right-sided colonic inflammation in patients with left-sided ulcerative chronic colitis. Inflammatory Bowel Diseases. 2004;**10**:215-219. DOI: 10.1097/00054725-200405000-00006

[15] Odze R. Diagnostic problems and advances in inflammatory bowel disease. Modern Pathology. 2003;**16**:348-358. DOI: 10.1097/01.MP.0000064746.82024.D1

[16] Bousvaros A, Antonioli DA, Colletti RB, Dubinsky MC, Glickman JN, Gold BD, et al. Differentiating ulcerative colitis from Crohn disease in children and young adults: Report of a working group of the North American Society for Pediatric Gastroenterology, Hepatology, and Nutrition and the Crohn's and Colitis Foundation of America. Journal of Pediatric Gastroenterology and Nutrition. 2007;**44**:653-674. DOI: 10.1097/MPG.0b013e31805563f3

[17] Lamb CA, Kennedy NA, Raine T, Hendy PA, Smith PJ, Limdi JK, et al. British Society of Gastroenterology consensus guidelines on the management of inflammatory bowel disease in adults. Gut. 2019;**68**:S1-S106. DOI: 10.1136/gutjnl-2019-318484

[18] Langner C, Magro F, Driessen A, Ensari A, Mantzaris GJ, Villanacci V, et al. The histopathological approach to inflammatory bowel disease: A practice guide. Virchows Archiv. 2014;**464**:511-527. DOI: 10.1007/s00428-014-1543-4

[19] Robert ME, Tang L, Hao LM, Reyes-Mugica M. Patterns of inflammation in mucosal biopsies of ulcerative colitis: perceived differences in pediatric populations are limited to children younger than 10 years. American Journal of Surgical Pathology. 2004;**28**:653-674. DOI: 10.1097/00000478-200402000-00005

[20] Swan NC, Geoghegan JG, O'Donoghue DP, Hyland JMP, Sheahan K. Fulminant colitis in inflammatory bowel disease: Detailed pathologic and clinical analysis. Diseases of the Colon and Rectum. 1998;**41**:1511-1515. DOI: 10.1007/BF02237298

[21] DeRoche TC, Xiao SY, Liu X. Histological evaluation in ulcerative colitis. Gastroenterology Report. 2014;**2**:178-192. DOI: 10.1093/gastro/gou031. Epub 2014 Jun 18

[22] Yantiss RK, Odze RD. Diagnostic difficulties in inflammatory bowel disease pathology. Histopathology. 2006;**48**:116-132. DOI: 10.1111/j.1365-2559.2005.02248.x

[23] Mosli MH, Parker CE, Nelson SA, Baker KA, Macdonald JK, Zou GY, et al. Histologic scoring indices for evaluation of disease activity in ulcerative colitis. Cochrane Database of Systematic Reviews. 2017;**2017**:1-34. DOI: 10.1002/14651858.CD011256.pub2

[24] Geboes K, Riddell R, Öst A, Jensfelt B, Persson T, Löfberg R. A reproducible grading scale for histological assessment of inflammation in ulcerative colitis. Gut. 2000;**47**:404-409. DOI: 10.1136/gut.47.3.404

[25] Magro F, Alves C, Lopes J, Lopes S, Tavares de Sousa H, Cotter J, et al. Histologic features of colon biopsies (Geboes score) associated with progression of ulcerative colitis for the first 36 months after biopsy. Clinical Gastroenterology and Hepatology. 2021;**19**:2567-2576. DOI: 10.1016/j.cgh.2020.09.017

[26] Marchal-Bressenot A, Salleron J, Boulagnon-Rombi C, Bastien C, Cahn V, Cadiot G, et al. Development and validation of the Nancy histological index for UC. Gut. 2017;**66**:43-49. DOI: 10.1136/gutjnl-2015-310187

[27] Mosli MH, Feagan BG, Zou G, Sandborn WJ, D'Haens G, Khanna R, et al. Development and validation of a histological index for UC. Gut. 2017;**66**:50-58. DOI: 10.1136/gutjnl-2015-310393

[28] MedMadonsa RDK, Mahendra BAGG, Silva H, Jayathunga DNU, Fernando J, Ediriweera DS, et al. Manchester Pathology 2021. 13th Joint Meeting of the British Division of the International Academy of Pathology and the Pathological Society of Great Britain &; Ireland, 6-8 July 2021. The Journal of Pathology. 2021;**255**:S1-S54. DOI: 10.1002/path.5793

[29] Odze RD, Harpaz N. Inflammtory bowel disease associated colorectal dysplasia. In: WHO Classification of Tumours Editorial Board, editor. WHO Classification of Tumours: Digestive System Tumours. 5th ed. Vol. 1. Lyon, France: IARC Publications; 2019. pp. 174-176

[30] Riddell RH, Goldman H, Ransohoff DF, Appelman HD, Fenoglio CM, Haggitt RC, et al. Dysplasia in inflammatory bowel disease: Standardized classification with provisional clinical applications. Human Pathology. 1983;**14**:931-969. DOI: 10.1016/S0046-8177(83)80175-0

[31] Schlemper RJ, Riddell RH, Kato Y, Borchard F, Cooper HS, Dawsey SM, et al. The vienna classification of gastrointestinal epithelial neoplasia. Gut. 2000;**47**:251-255. DOI: 10.1136/gut.47.2.251

[32] Lichtiger S, Present DH, Kornbluth A, Gelernt I, Bauer J, Galler G, et al. Cyclosporine in severe ulcerative colitis refractory to steroid therapy. New England Journal of Medicine. 1994;**330**:1841-1845. DOI: 10.1056/nejm199406303302601

[33] Laine L, Kaltenbach T, Barkun A, McQuaid KR, Subramanian V, Soetikno R. SCENIC international consensus statement on surveillance and management of dysplasia in inflammatory bowel disease. Gastroenterology. 2015;**148**:639-651. DOI: 10.1053/j.gastro.2015.01.031

Section 4

Special Population

Chapter 6

Pediatric Ulcerative Colitis

Rayna Shentova-Eneva and Ivan Yankov

Abstract

Inflammatory bowel disease (IBD) is a collective term that includes a group of disorders with unknown etiology characterized by chronic inflammation of the gastrointestinal tract and relapsing and remitting course. Ulcerative colitis (UC) is a type of IBD that affects the large intestine, causing irritation, inflammation, and ulcers in its lining. Approximately 25% of patients with IBD are diagnosed before the age of 18 years. Children and adolescents with UC are more likely to have more severe disease course with more extended intestinal involvement at diagnosis and faster disease progression than adults. Atypical presentation is also common in pediatric age. Treatment recommendations for children and adolescents are different than those for adults and offer many unique challenges for the healthcare professionals.

Keywords: typical ulcerative colitis, atypical ulcerative colitis, severe ulcerative colitis, diagnostic approach, management of pediatric ulcerative colitis

1. Introduction

Inflammatory bowel disease (IBD) represents a group of chronic disorders of the digestive tract with a relapsing and remitting clinical course and a debilitating character. IBD may occur at any age [1]. Approximately 25% of incident cases of inflammatory bowel disease occur during childhood [2–4]. The majority of newly diagnosed pediatric patients are teenagers, but the disease may have an earlier manifestation [5, 6]. According to the Montreal classification of IBD the pediatric IBD (PIBD) is defined as having an age of occurrence younger than 17 years [7]. Later the Paris classification defined A1a group for those children with less than 10 years of age IBD onset and A1b for children with onset of symptoms between 10 and <17 years of age [8]. The latest modification of the IBD classification defines disease onset under the age of 17 as PIBD and this is further classified into early onset IBD (EOIBD) when it occurs under 10 years of age, very early onset IBD (VEOIBD) with less than 6 years of age IBD onset, infantile (and toddler) onset of IBD (less than 2 years of onset) and neonatal IBD (disease onset within first 28 days of age) [9].

Evidence over the last several years have shown that VEOIBD is a separate disease entity with specific clinical features and outcomes that are different from those of adolescent-onset IBD [9, 10]. In most cases VEOIBD is associated with underlying primary immunodeficiencies or has an underlying monogenic etiology. It is characterized by a severe and often treatment-refractory course of disease [11]. Not surprisingly VEOIBD is accepted currently as a unique disease that requires a specific diagnostic approach and specific treatment. A recent position paper summarized the diagnostic algorithm by suspected VEOIBD and described some of the potential treatments [12].

The classically group of IBDs in childhood includes three nosological entities: Crohn's disease (CD), IBD-unclassified (IBDU) and ulcerative colitis (UC) and [13].

CD is a type of IBD whose predilection site for development is the terminal ileum, but it may affect any part of the gastrointestinal tract, from the mouth to the anus [14]. The changes are usually segmental, the diseased sections alternating with healthy ones—the so-called skip lesions. The inflammation in CD is transmural and may affect the entire bowel wall. Initially, infiltrates are localized around the intestinal crypts, but with the disease progression, deeper layers are involved, and specific histological structures are formed—non-caseating epithelioid granulomas [13–16]. The transmural inflammation predetermines the disease-specific complications: wall thickening and narrowing of the lumen of the intestine, intestinal obstruction, fistulation, and abscess formation [16].

IBDU is the rarest of the IBD subgroups. It is more common in the pediatric population than in adults and is a diagnosis which is made in patients with IBD in whom the inflammation is confined to the colon and the disease has characteristics which do not allow to determine definitively whether it is UC or CD despite all necessary tests [7, 13, 16–18].

In UC, the inflammatory changes are usually localized in the colonic mucosa. The inflammation is ulcerative and purulent. It is continuous, usually starting from the rectum and gradually extending to the more proximal parts of the bowel. Histological findings include chronic inflammation of the mucosa with infiltration of polymorphonuclear neutrophils, accumulation of polymorphonuclear neutrophils in the crypts of the large intestine, formation of crypt abscesses, and disruption of the structure of the mucous glands. In more severe cases, inflammatory pseudopolyps are formed. The wall of the intestine becomes thick and rigid, without haustration [5, 6, 11, 13, 14, 16].

2. Specific features of pediatric ulcerative colitis

Pediatric ulcerative colitis is a different disease entity from adult-onset UC. It has a particular etiopathogenesis, unique clinical characteristics, specific disease course and outcome.

2.1 Etiopathogenesis

The etiopathogenesis of IBD is complex and multifactorial. It is suggested that a dysregulation of mucosal immune system leads to excessive inflammatory response to the contents of the intestinal lumen (microflora, infectious agents, nutrients, etc.). This abnormal immune response results in chronic inflammation and damaging of body's own structures [20]. Different genetic and environmental factors may contribute to the development of the immune dysregulation and the abnormal immune response [21]. Typical for the pathogenesis of pediatric IBD is that the role of the genetic factors is stronger than in adults, while environmental factors are of major importance in later clinical manifestation [22–24].

Childhood-onset UC is often associated with a consanguinity and a positive family history of IBD which provides an additional clue to an underlying genetic predisposition [25].

Currently, over genetic 160 loci have been associated with IBD. Most of the variants lead to aberrations in several mechanisms altering the intestinal immune homeostasis and contribute to both CD and UC risk. However, some polymorphisms are unique to UC- or early-onset UC-specific risk [26–28]. Furthermore, some types of infantile IBD or VEOIBD that manifest phenotypically with UC are thought to be monogenic diseases having a Mendelian inheritance [9, 12].

2.2 Clinical manifestation

The most common symptoms of pediatric UC include abdominal pain, chronic diarrhea with or without blood, weight loss, fatigue, fever, and rectorrhagia [6]. Generally, the clinical manifestation of the disease is associated with its location and the degree of inflammation [29]. Children with UC have more extended disease compared to adults with UC [30]. They are likely to present with pancolitis, whereas in adults the disease is predominantly confined to the rectum or left side of the colon [16]. The differences in disease location result in different clinical presentation in comparison with adult patients with UC. The majority of children with UC report of abdominal pain and bloody diarrhea, whereas adults tend to present most often with rectal bleeding [14, 16]. Furthermore, pediatric patients with UC have more often extraintestinal manifestations, impaired nutritional status or are at impaired general condition compared to adults with UC [30–32].

2.3 Endoscopic findings

The typical endoscopic findings of UC are continuous mucosal inflammation that starts from the rectum, extends proximally, and ends at transition zone anywhere in the colon or involves the whole colon [13]. Sometimes, in case of severe pancolitis the ileocecal valve and the most distal part of the terminal ileum may also be affected. This extension of the inflammatory process is termed "backwash ileitis" [14]. The typical macroscopic features of UC include erythema, granularity, friability, purulent exudates and ulcers which usually appear as superficial small ulcers. The typical histologic findings of UC include chronic inflammation in the mucosa accompanied by cryptitis or crypt abscesses. The inflammation is most severe distally and is getting milder proximally [13].

Pediatric-onset UC may present also with atypical endoscopic findings. Recognized and described are the following 5 phenotypes [13, 19]:

1. **Rectal sparing UC:** 5–30% of pediatric patients with UC have reduced or no inflammation of the rectum compared to proximal colon.

2. **Short duration of disease**: This variant occurs primarily in children younger than 10 years of age and is characterized by patchy disease in biopsies or lack of typical architectural distortion in pathological specimens.

3. **Cecal patch:** This phenotype is observed in 2% of the pediatric patients with UC and is characterized by left sided colitis with an area of cecal inflammation

4. **Involvement of the upper gastrointestinal tract:** 4–8% of the children with UC present with mild ulceration and microscopic involvement of the stomach; 0.8% of them present with inflammatory changes in the esophagus or duodenum—usually erosions, rarely ulcerations.

5. **Acute severe UC:** Children with clinical manifestation of acute severe ulcerative colitis may have several features that are typically characteristic of CD such as transmural inflammation and deep ulcers, which are associated with the severity of the disease.

Based on the specific endoscopic manifestations of pediatric UC in 2013 was introduced the term "atypical UC": a new child-specific IBD category consisting of 5 atypical disease phenotypes. Nowadays the pediatric UC is divided into typical UC and atypical UC [13].

2.4 Evolution and outcome

In contrast to adult-onset presentations, children with UC have extended disease and are likely to present with pancolitis [26, 33]. This more extended disease is consistently associated with a more severe and aggressive disease course. According to the literature, within 5 years from diagnosis a significantly higher percentage of patients with childhood-onset UC are admitted to emergency units for acute severe colitis, compared to adult-onset disease [33]. Furthermore, children with UC are more likely to receive corticosteroids, be initiated on immunomodulators, and require surgery in the first year after diagnosis than adults with UC [26, 33].

The colectomy rate is significantly higher in children compared to adult UC populations [33]. Based on the literature the colectomy rate within 10 years from diagnosis is over 40% in pediatric-onset UC compared to less than 20% in adult-onset UC [34]. However, other studies show lower colectomy rates of 25% in 6 years and 15% in 10 years [35, 36].

Another specific feature of childhood-onset UC is the possible change in the diagnosis from onset to long-term follow-up [6]. A recent study of the natural history of pediatric-onset IBD showed an increased disease reclassification over time from UC diagnosis to CD diagnosis [37]. Patients initially diagnosed as UC (a correct initial diagnosis) developed findings that led to a diagnostic change to CD [38].

3. Classification of pediatric ulcerative colitis

In May 2009 an international group of experts in pediatric IBD met in Paris and created a classification which reflects the specific phenotypic characteristics of pediatric IBD—the so-called Paris classification (**Table 1**). It represents a pediatric modification of the adult Montreal Classification of IBD. The classification of pediatric UC disease according to the Paris classification. With respect to disease extent it is divided into four categories: ulcerative proctitis (E1), left-sided UC (E2), extensive UC (E3) and pancolitis (E4). Disease severity is categorized as never severe (S0) and ever severe (S1) [8].

Extent of disease			
E1	**E2**	**E3**	**E4**
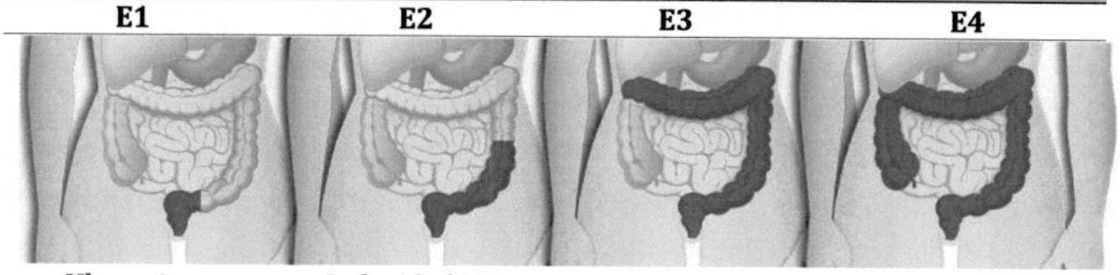			
Ulcerative proctitis	Left-sided UC (distal to splenic flexure)	Extensive (hepatic flexure distally)	Pancolitis (proximal to hepatic flexure)
Severity of disease			
S0 Never severe (never PUCAI≥65)		**S1** Ever severe (ever PUCAI≥65)	

PUCAI: Pediatric Ulcerative Colitis Activity Index

Table 1.
Paris classifications for pediatric ulcerative colitis (adapted from Levine et al. [8]).

For measuring disease activity and evaluation of disease severity is used a validated, multi-item, scoring system—the so-called Pediatric Ulcerative Colitis Activity Index (PUCAI) (**Table 2**). The PUCAI is a score comprised of six parameters, including the assessment of abdominal pain, rectal bleeding, stool consistency, number of stools per 24 h, nocturnal stools, and activity level. Each item is assigned a value contributing to a combined total PUCAI score ranging from 0 to 85. Categories of UC disease activity are defined by the following total PUCAI scores: 0–9 (no activity), 10–34 (mild activity), 35–64 (moderate activity), and 65–85 (severe activity) [39]. The items that are included in the PUCAI score and their corresponding points are presented.

Item	Characteristics	Points
Abdominal pain	No pain	0
	Pain can be ignored	5
	Pain cannot be ignored	10
Rectal bleeding	None	0
	Small amount only, in less than 50% of stools	10
	Small amount with most stools	20
	Large amount (>50% of the stool content)	30
Stool consistency of most stools	Formed	0
	Partially formed	5
	Completely unformed	10
Number of stools per 24 h	0–2	0
	3–5	5
	6–8	10
	>8	15
Nocturnal stools (any episode causing wakening)	No	0
	Yes	10
Activity level	No limitation of activity	0
	Occasional limitation of activity	5
	Severe restricted activity	10
Total score:		

Table 2.
Pediatric ulcerative colitis activity index (adapted from Turner et al. [39]).

4. Diagnosis of pediatric ulcerative colitis

The diagnosis of pediatric UC is based on standard consensus-based criteria for diagnosing IBD in pediatric patients, the so-called Porto criteria. They were prepared and issued in 2005 by the IBD Working Group of the European Society for Pediatric Gastroenterology, Hepatology and Nutrition [16]. In 2013 the initial criteria were revised and updated [13]. According to the Porto criteria the diagnosis of pediatric UC involves history taking, physical and laboratory examination, esophagogastroduodenoscopy and ileocolonoscopy with histology, and imaging of the small bowel [11, 13, 16]:

1. **History:** Abdominal pain and bloody diarrhea are the most common presenting symptoms in pediatric UC. Other symptoms may be rectal bleeding, fever, weight loss, growth retardation, malnutrition, psychiatric symptoms, arthropathy, erythema nodosum, retardation of pubertal development, secondary amenorrhea, etc. Suspicious are symptoms which persist for ≥4 weeks or recurrent symptoms (≥2 episodes within 6 months).

2. **Physical examination:** Physical examination might reveal signs of anemia, abdominal tenderness, and blood on rectal exam. Looking for presence of malnutrition or extraintestinal manifestations (skin abnormalities, arthritis, etc.) is an important part of the full examination.

3. **Blood tests:** Screening blood tests should include full blood count, erythrocyte sedimentation rate, C-reactive protein, serum levels of urea and creatinine, serum albumin, immunoelectrophoresis, liver function tests and (in certain cases) celiac screen.

4. **Microbiological investigations:** The search for bacterial infections should include a stool culture to exclude Samonella, Shigella, Yersinia, Campylobacter as well as *Clostridum difficile* toxins in all children.

5. **Screening for tuberculosis**

6. **Serological investigations:** No serology pattern can preclude the diagnosis of UC, due to imperfect test performance of all existing antibodies. However, the presence of pANCA+/ASCA- serology increases the likelihood of UC.

7. **Fecal markers of inflammation:** Pediatric data exist primarily for fecal calprotectin and lactoferrin. Both markers are excellent tools for identifying the presence of intestinal inflammation but are unspecific.

8. **Ileocolonoscopy and esophagogastroduodenoscopy with biopsies:** Colonoscopy including intubation of the terminal ileum and multiple biopsies for histology obtained from all segments of the lower intestinal tract (ileum, cecum, ascending colon, transverse colon, descending colon, sigmoid and rectum) is essential for the diagnosis of pediatric UC. In addition, an esophagogastroduodenoscopy is advocated is recommended in all patients to exclude a CD or to confirm an atypical UC.

9. **Imaging of the small bowel:** It is recommended for all patients unless the diagnosis favors typical UC. **Magnetic resonance enterography** is the imaging modality

of choice in children IBD at diagnosis with high diagnostic accuracy. Alternatively, **wireless capsule endoscopy** can be used to identify small bowel mucosal lesions in children in whom magnetic resonance enterography cannot be performed. **Abdominal ultrasound** is also a useful imaging modality that accurately detects and characterizes inflammation of the bowel wall, but it is more valuable in CD diagnosis and usually should be complemented by more sensitive imaging method.

10. **Genetic tests and immunological investigations:** They are recommended for all patients with suspected VEOIBD, presenting with UC phenotype.

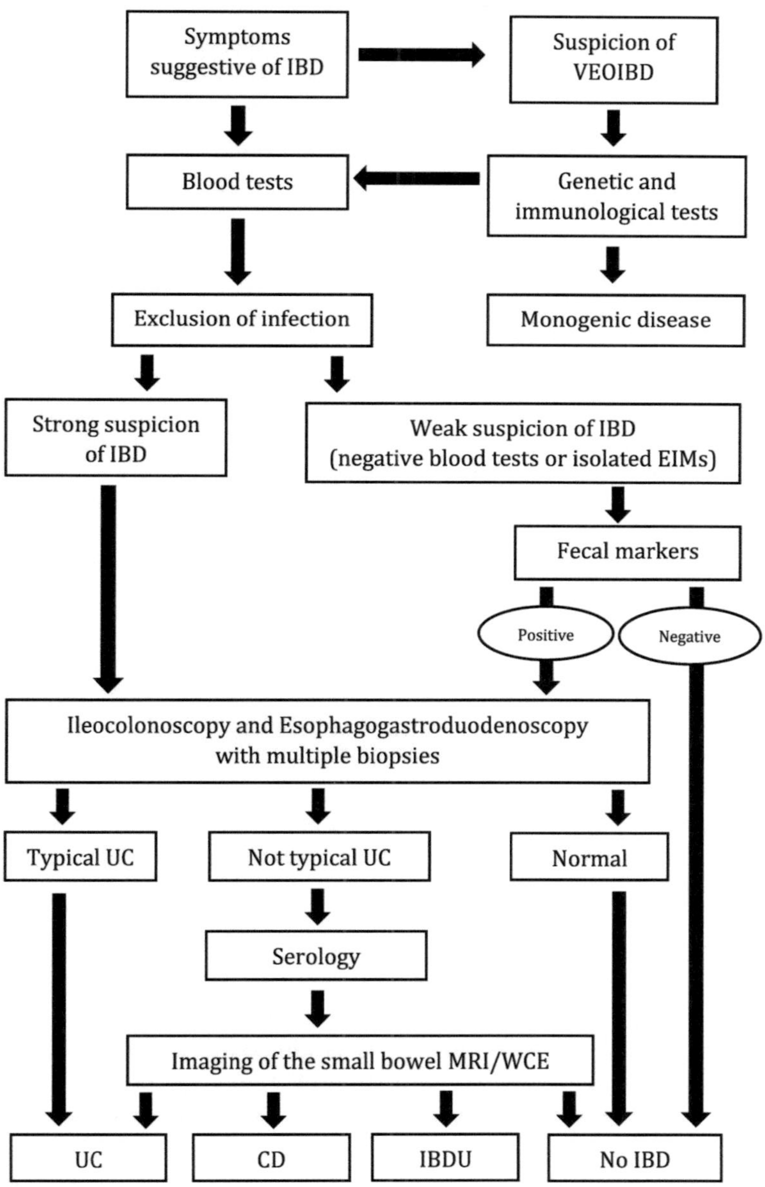

Figure 1.
Diagnostic algorithm for pediatric ulcerative colitis. IBD: inflammatory bowel disease; VEOIBD: very early onset inflammatory bowel disease; EIM: extraintestinal manifestation; UC: ulcerative colitis; MRI: magnetic resonance imaging; WCE: wireless capsule endoscopy; CD: Crohn's disease; IBDU: Inflammatory bowel disease unclassified.

A summary of the diagnostic algorithm for suspected pediatric UC is presented at **Figure 1**.

5. Therapy of pediatric ulcerative colitis

The management of pediatric UC is based on therapeutic guidelines produced by the European Crohn's and Colitis Organization (ECCO) and European Society for Pediatric Gastroenterology Hepatology and Nutrition (ESPGHAN) [40, 41]. Generally, the treatment strategy should be guided by the endoscopic extent of inflammation and disease severity. However, in children with UC the therapy depends mainly on disease severity, assessed by the corresponding disease activity index: Pediatric Ulcerative Colitis Activity Index (PUCAI) [39, 40]. The treatment goal is induction and maintenance of steroid-free complete remission [40].

5.1 Medical therapy

5.1.1 5-Aminosalicylates (5-ASA)

5-ASA are the preferred first-line therapy for induction and maintenance of remission for patients with mild (PUCAI 10–34) and some patients with moderate disease (PUCAI 35–64) [40]. The preparations are available as forms for local administration (suppositories and enemas) and forms for systemic administration (tablets and granules). Topical 5-ASA are effective in mild-to-moderate distal UC, but usually they are combined with oral 5-ASA, as the combination therapy is more effective than either treatment alone [40, 42]. Rectal 5-ASA are superior to rectal steroids for induction and maintenance of remission in distal UC [43]. Oral 5-ASA preparations are generally preferred to sulfasalazine due to a superior side effect profile combined with similar efficacy. However, sulfasalazine is cheaper and available in liquid formulation [40, 42]. The recommended dosing for oral mesalamine is 60–80 mg/kg/day (maximum 4.8 g daily) and for oral sulfasalazine 40–70 mg/kg/day (maximum 4 g daily). Both are usually given in divided doses, but according to the studies once daily dosing of 5-ASA may be as effective as twice daily dosing [44]. The recommended dosing for rectal mesalamine is 25 mg/kg up to 1 g daily (1 g daily is as effective as higher doses) [40]. Lack of meaningful response to 5-ASA within 2–3 weeks of therapy is an indication for treatment modification and initiation of steroids [40, 42].

5.1.2 Steroids

Treatment with steroids is recommended for induction of remission in children with moderate and severe UC. It is not recommended for maintenance of remission [40]. Available are forms for oral, intravenous, and local administration. Steroid dependency is defined as response or remission with corticosteroid treatment, but recurrence of symptoms when the dose is lowered or within 3 months following complete taper [40]. Steroid refractory UC is defined as lack of clinical response to oral prednisolone at doses 0.75–1 mg/kg/day (max. 40 mg/day) within 4 weeks or lack of clinical response to intravenous prednisolone at doses 0.75–1 mg/kg/day (max. 60 mg/day) within 1 week [40, 41].

Oral steroids should be used as second-line therapy for mild or moderate UC not responding to 5-ASA (oral ± rectal) and may be considered as first line in more severe moderate disease. The recommended daily dose for oral prednisolone/prednisone is 1 mg/kg/day up to 40 mg/day administered once daily (in the morning) for 2–3 weeks followed by a tapering period of up to 8–10 weeks [40]. Second-generation oral steroids with lower systemic effect such as beclomethasone dipropionate and budesonide-MMX may be considered in patients with mild disease refractory to 5-ASA before oral prednisolone. The recommended dosing schedule for beclomethasone dipropionate is 5 mg once daily for 4 weeks and for budesonide-MMX 9 mg for 8 weeks. The recommendations are for patients with weight > 30 kg. Dosing for children <30 kg has not been established [40].

Intravenous steroids should be used as first-line therapy in patients with severe UC (PUCAI ≥ 65) (See section Acute severe ulcerative colitis) [40, 41].

Rectal steroid preparations are useful for patients who are 5-ASA intolerant and in selected patients refractory to 5-ASA before starting oral prednisolone [40].

5.1.3 Immunomodulators

Thiopurines are recommended for maintaining remission in children with UC. They should be used as second-line therapy for maintaining remission in children with mild or moderate UC after 5-ASA failed and as first-line therapy for maintaining remission in children with severe UC and in 5-ASA intolerant patients. Although thiopurines have been shown to be more effective than 5-ASA they should generally be reserved as second-line therapy, considering their safety profile [40]. Before starting therapy with thiopurines it is recommended the determination of thiopurines methyltransferase (TPMT) genotype or phenotype to identify patients at greater risk of early profound myelosuppression or other thiopurine associated toxicity. Dose should be reduced in heterozygous patients or in those with low activity. Thiopurines should not be used in children homozygous mutants for TPMT or those with very low TPMT activity. Concomitant use of allopurinol 50 mg once daily in patients <30 kg and 100 mg once daily in patients ≥30 kg (maximum 5 mg/kg) with reduced dose of azathioprine (to approximately 25–30% of initial dose) is a valid therapeutic option in cases of hyperactive TPMT resulting in high 6-MMP and low 6-TGN. The recommended dosing in patients with normal TPMT is 2–2.5 mg/kg/day for azathioprine and 1–1.5 mg/kg/day for mercaptopurine, in a single daily dose [40]. The therapeutic effect of thiopurines may take up to 10–14 weeks after the start of treatment. Measurement of thiopurine metabolites, 6-methyl mercaptopurine and 6-thioguanine is helpful to assess compliance, adjust therapy and avoid adverse events [40, 42].

Methotrexate may be considered as alternative therapeutic option for maintaining remission in selected children with UC. Generally, there is no evidence supporting its routine use for maintenance of remission in UC, therefore it should be used only when other alternatives are not possible or available [40, 45].

Tacrolimus is a potent immunomodulator which administration is reserved for special occasions. Oral tacrolimus may be considered in selected outpatient UC children as another option to steroids for bridging to thiopurines or vedolizumab. The target trough level should be 10–15 ng/mL when initiating the treatment, and 5–10 ng/mL during the follow up period. Rectal tacrolimus may be considered as third-line therapy in patients with ulcerative proctitis who are either refractory or intolerant to mesalamine and steroids topical therapies. The recommended dose is 0.07 mg/kg/day, maximum 3 mg/day [40].

5.1.4 Biologics

Treatment with biologics is recommended as second- or third-line therapy for children with moderate or severe UC. Currently approved for pediatric use are three tumor necrosis factor (TNF)-alpha inhibitors: *infliximab*, *adalimumab*, *golimumab*; and one anti-integrin drug: *vedolizumab*. However, the mainstay of pediatric UC management is the therapy with *infliximab*. It is used for induction and maintenance of remission in children and adolescents who have had an inadequate response to conventional therapy including corticosteroids and thiopurines or who are intolerant to or have medical contraindications for such therapies. The recommended dose is 5 mg/kg per dose at weeks 0, 2, and 6, then 5 mg/kg every 8 weeks thereafter. Higher dosing should be considered in children with low body weight (<30 kg) or high BMI, and in the presence of higher inflammatory burden and hypoalbuminemia. A combination therapy with immunomodulator is preferred to reduce the likelihood of developing drug-antibodies and to enhance the effectiveness [40]. Target trough levels during induction are ≥15 μg/mL and post induction at the start of maintenance (week 14) ≥5 μg/mL [46–48].

Adalimumab or *golimumab* may be considered as therapeutic option in children with moderate to severe UC who are intolerant to *infliximab* or initially respond but then lose response to *infliximab* (secondary loss of response). The recommended dosing for *adalimumab* is 160 mg at week 0, followed by 80 mg after 2 weeks and then 40 mg every other week in adolescents with weight ≥ 40 kg. In children with weight < 40 kg the recommended dosing is 92 mg/m^2 at week 0, followed by 46 mg/m^2 after 2 weeks and then 23 mg/m^2 every other week. *Adalimumab* target levels should be ≥13 μg/mL during the induction phase and ≥7.5 μg/mL during the maintenance phase [47, 49]. The recommended dosing for *golimumab* is 200 mg at week 0 followed by 100 mg at week 2 and every 4 weeks thereafter in adolescents with weight ≥ 45 kg. In children with weight < 45 kg the recommended dosing is 115 mg/m^2 at week 0, followed by 60 mg/m^2 at week 2 and every 4 weeks thereafter. Recommended target trough levels during maintenance are >2 mg/mL [40].

5.1.5 Antibiotics

Antibiotics should not be routinely used for induction or maintenance of remission of pediatric [40]. However, recent studies demonstrated that a combination of specific antibiotics—the so called wide-spectrum antibiotic cocktail could be used as therapeutic option for pediatric patients with severe UC resistant to other treatments [50, 51].

5.1.6 Probiotics

The use of specific probiotic agents (e.g., VSL#3 or *Escherichia coli* Nissle 917) may be considered as an adjuvant therapy in pediatric patients with mild UC or as first-line therapy in selected patients with mild UC intolerant to 5-ASA [40].

5.2 Surgical therapy

Despite advances in conventional therapy surgery remains an integral part of the management strategy in children with UC. It should be considered in patients with active, or steroid-dependent, UC despite optimized medical therapy, and in those with colon dysplasia [40]. The most common surgery that is carried out is a subtotal/total colectomy with a temporary stoma [42]. A minimally invasive laparoscopic approach is recommended for superior outcomes. Generally, the restorative proctocolectomy with ileal pouch-anal anastomosis and a covering loop ileostomy, performed as one- or two- or three-stage procedures is the recommended elective surgery for pediatric patients with UC [40].

5.3 Acute severe ulcerative colitis

Acute severe ulcerative colitis (ASC) is defined by a PUCAI score of at least 65 points [39]. According to the literature 11–23% of children with UC experience at least one severe exacerbation during the course of their disease [52–54]. ASC is an emergency which requires immediate management. Children with ASC should be treated in a hospital by a multidisciplinary team. They need close monitoring and frequent reevaluation [41].

Intravenous methylprednisolone is used as first-line treatment for ASC in children. It is preferred over hydrocortisone due to its minimal mineralocorticoid activity. The recommended dosage is 1–1.5 mg/kg/day (up to 60 mg/day) given in one or two divided daily doses. The majority of patients will respond to this treatment. However, sequential measurement of PUCAI scores is essential for identifying those patients requiring a step up in treatment with second-line (rescue) therapy [41, 42]. A PUCAI score of >45 on day 3 indicated a likelihood of steroid failure and should dictate planning for second-line therapy. In children with a PUCAI of 35–65 on day 5 intravenous steroids should be continued for an additional 2–5 days before a decision on second-line therapy is made. A PUCAI score of >65 on day 5 indicated the need for starting a rescue therapy [41].

The second-line therapy involves either *infliximab* or calcineurin inhibitors (*cyclosporin* or *tacrolimus*) [41]. Both are equally effective in inducing clinical remission in children with ASC [55]. Due to increased clearance of *infliximab* in ASC the recommended dosing for induction of remission is higher up to 10 mg/kg per dose and may be given more frequently than usual (e.g., weeks 0, 1, and 4–5). After achievement of remission target drug levels should be 5–10 μg/mL. The recommended dosage for *tacrolimus* is 0.1 mg/kg per dose orally twice daily with target drug levels during induction 10–15 ng/mL and 5–7 ng/mL once remission achieved. The recommended induction dosage for *cyclosporine* is 2 mg/kg/day administered as continuous intravenous infusion. Target drug levels should be 150–300 ng/mL during the induction phase and 100–200 ng/mL during the maintenance phase. Response to rescue therapy should be judged daily by PUCAI. If the rescue therapy fails, there is an option for a second-line rescue therapy in selected patients or it should be proceeded to a surgical management [41].

Many gastrointestinal infections have been associated with pediatric ASC. Exclusion of several specific pathogens, such as *Clostridium difficile* or Cytomegalovirus is crucial for the adequate management. In addition, for all patients on triple immunosuppressive therapy which includes *anti-TNF* or a calcineurin inhibitor plus *thiopurines* or *methotrexate* plus steroids should be considered a *Pneumocystis jiroveci* pneumonia prophylaxis with *trimethoprim-sulfamethoxazole*. The recommended trimethoprim-sulfamethoxazole dosing is 450 mg/m^2 twice daily (maximum 1.92 g daily) for 3 days each week, either consecutive or alternate day dosing [41].

ASC is associated with increased risk for venous thromboembolic events (VTE) [56–58]. However, thromboprophylaxis with subcutaneous low molecular weight heparin is recommended only for children or adolescents with an underlying predisposition such as smoking, use of oral contraceptives, complete immobilization, obesity, concurrent significant infection, known prothrombotic disorder, previous VTE, family history of VTE, etc. [41].

Adequate nutrient intake and early treatment of the accompanying conditions such as anemia, infections, etc., are also an integral part of the successful management of ASC and should not be overlooked.

5.4 Very early onset inflammatory bowel disease with colitis phenotype

The colitis phenotype is the most common in the VEOIBD group [40]. The clinical manifestation could be very heterogeneous and requires a different treatment approach altogether [12]. A large percentage of children with VEOIBD presenting as colitis have a mild disease which can be easily managed with 5-ASA [59]. Others demonstrate an extended disease with severe and treatment refractory course. They require escalated dosing strategies and more intensive treatments: early introduction of biologics, combination therapies, higher dosage of immunomodulators or biologics, etc. [12]. Additionally, many of the patients with VEOIBD with colitis phenotype have an underlying monogenic disorder and benefit from specific targeted therapies [12, 40]. If the molecular defect is caused by a mutation affecting predominantly immunological cells (e.g., IL10 signaling defects, XIAP and chronic granulomatous disease), hematopoietic stem cell transplantation may be curative [40]. Therapies that inhibit the hyperactive T-cell signaling could be used successfully in patients with *CTLA4* or *LRBA* defects [60]. *Abatacept* and *rapamycin* could also be used in those patients and in patients with other defects that involve loss of Tregs or unchecked T-cell activation, such as *FOXP3* and *PIK3CD* mutations. Generally, targeted medical therapies can be used in a variety of monogenic diseases as a maintenance therapy, and in some cases, as a bridge to hematopoietic stem cell transplantation [12].

6. Conclusions

Pediatric UC is a disease with a heterogeneous phenotype which poses many unique challenges. The majority of children with UC present with pancolitis. Since disease extent is consistently associated with disease severity, it is not surprising that they have more aggressive disease course requiring more intensive therapies. Furthermore, children with UC have some unique age-related issues, such as delay of growth and pubertal development, nutrition disorders, psychological or emotional problems. Pediatric UC may present also atypically making the diagnosis difficult and demanding specific diagnostic tests and procedures. In addition, there is a group of patients with early-onset UC who needs a completely different diagnostic and treatment approach.

Pediatric UC is a disease with unique features and characteristics. Its correct diagnosis and successful management always require a hard teamwork and multidisciplinary approach.

Conflict of interest

The authors declare no conflict of interest.

DOI: http://dx.doi.org/10.5772/intechopen.102226

Author details

Rayna Shentova-Eneva[1,2*] and Ivan Yankov[3,4]

1 Department of Gastroenterology and Hepatology, University Children's Hospital "Prof. Ivan Mitev", Sofia, Bulgaria

2 Medical University of Sofia, Bulgaria

3 Department of Pediatrics and Medical Genetics, University Hospital "St. George", Plovdiv, Bulgaria

4 Medical University of Plovdiv, Bulgaria

*Address all correspondence to: rshentova@yahoo.com

References

[1] Duricova D, Burisch J, Jess T, Gower-Rousseau C, Lakatos PL. Age-related differences in presentation and course of inflammatory bowel disease: An update on the population-based literature. Journal of Crohn's & Colitis. 2014;**8**:1351-1361. DOI: 10.1016/j.crohns.2014.05.006

[2] Auvin S, Molinié F, Gower-Rousseau C, Brazier F, Merle V, et al. Incidence, clinical presentation and location at diagnosis of pediatric infl ammatory bowel disease: A prospective population-based study in northern France (1988-1999). Journal of Pediatric Gastroenterology and Nutrition. 2005;**41**:49-55

[3] Baldassano RN, Piccoli DA. Inflammatory bowel disease in pediatric and adolescent patients. Gastroenterology Clinics of North America. 1999;**28**:445-458

[4] Braegger CP, Ballabeni P, Rogler D, Vavricka SR, Friedt M, et al. Epidemiology of inflammatory bowel disease: Is there a shift towards onset at a younger age? Journal of Pediatric Gastroenterology and Nutrition. 2011;**53**:141-144

[5] Heyman MB, Kirschner BS, Gold BD, Ferry G, Baldassano R, et al. Children with early onset inflammatory bowel disease (IBD): Analysis of a pediatric IBD consortium registry. The Journal of Pediatrics. 2005;**146**(1):35-40

[6] Mamula P, Telega GW, Markowitz JE, Brown KA, Russo PA, et al. Inflammatory bowel disease in children 5 years of age and younger. The American Journal of Gastroenterology. 2002;**97**:2005-2010

[7] Satsangi J, Silverberg MS, Vermeire S, Colombel JF. The Montreal classification of inflammatory bowel disease: Controversies, consensus, and implications. Gut. 2006;**55**:749-753. DOI: 10.1136/gut.2005.082909

[8] Levine A, Griffiths A, Markowitz J, Wilson DC, Turner D, et al. Pediatric modification of the Montreal classification for inflammatory bowel disease: The Paris classification. Inflammatory Bowel Diseases. 2011;**17**:1314-1321. DOI: 10.1002/ibd.21493

[9] Uhlig HH, Charbit-Henrion F, Kotlarz D, Shouval DS, Schwerd T, et al. Clinical genomics for the diagnosis of monogenic forms of inflammatory bowel disease: A position paper from the paediatric IBD Porto Group of European Society of Paediatric Gastroenterology, Hepatology and Nutrition. Journal of Pediatric Gastroenterology and Nutrition. 2021;**1**:456-473. DOI: 10.1097/MPG.0000000000003017

[10] Shim JO, Seo JK. Very early-onset inflammatory bowel disease (IBD) in infancy is a different disease entity from adult-onset IBD; one form of interleukin-10 receptor mutations. Journal of Human Genetics. 2014;**59**:337-341. DOI: 10.1038/jhg.2014.32

[11] Ouahed J, Spencer E, Kotlarz D, Shouval DS, Kowalik M, et al. Very early onset inflammatory bowel disease: A clinical approach with a focus on the role of genetics and underlying immune deficiencies. Inflammatory Bowel Diseases. 2020;**12**:820-842. DOI: 10.1093/ibd/izz259

[12] Kelsen JR, Sullivan KE, Rabizadeh S, Singh N, Snapper S, et al. North American Society for Pediatric

Gastroenterology, Hepatology, and Nutrition position paper on the evaluation and management for patients with very early-onset inflammatory bowel disease. Journal of Pediatric Gastroenterology and Nutrition. 2020;**70**:389-403. DOI: 10.1097/MPG.0000000000002567

[13] Levine A, Koletzko S, Turner D, Escher JC, Cucchiara S, et al. ESPGHAN revised porto criteria for the diagnosis of inflammatory bowel disease in children and adolescents. Journal of Pediatric Gastroenterology and Nutrition. 2014;**58**:795-806. DOI: 10.1097/MPG.0000000000000239

[14] Mamula P, Markowitz JE, Baldassano RN. Pediatric Inflammatory Bowel Disease. 2nd ed. New York, NY, USA: Springer; 2013

[15] de Bie CI, Buderus S, Sandhu BK, de Ridder L, Paerregaard A, et al. Diagnostic workup of paediatric patients with inflammatory bowel disease in Europe: Results of a 5-year audit of the EUROKIDS registry. Journal of Pediatric Gastroenterology and Nutrition. 2012;**54**:374-380. DOI: 10.1097/MPG.0b013e318231d984

[16] IBD Working Group of the European Society for Paediatric Gastroenterology, Hepatology and Nutrition. Inflammatory bowel disease in children and adolescents: Recommendations for diagnosis—the Porto criteria. Journal of Pediatric Gastroenterology and Nutrition. 2005;**41**:1-7. DOI: 10.1097/01.mpg.0000163736.30261.82

[17] Carvalho RS, Abadom V, Dilworth HP, Thompson R, Oliva-Hemker M, et al. Indeterminate colitis: A significant subgroup of pediatric IBD. Inflammatory Bowel Diseases. 2006;**12**:258-262. DOI: 10.1097/01.MIB.0000215093.62245.b9

[18] Lindberg E, Lindquist B, Holmquist L, Hildebrand H. Journal of Pediatric Gastroenterology and Nutrition;**2000**:30,259-30,264. DOI: 10.1097/00005176-200003000-00009

[19] Levine A, de Bie CI, Turner D, Cucchiara S, Sladek M, et al. Atypical disease phenotypes in pediatric ulcerative colitis: 5-year analyses of the EUROKIDS Registry. Inflammatory Bowel Diseases. 2013;**19**:370-377. DOI: 10.1002/ibd.23013

[20] Xu XR, Liu CQ, Feng BS, Liu ZJ. Dysregulation of mucosal immune response in pathogenesis of inflammatory bowel disease. World Journal of Gastroenterology. 2014;**20**:3255-3264. DOI: 10.3748/wjg.v20.i12.3255

[21] Khor B, Gardet A, Xavier RJ. Genetics and pathogenesis of inflammatory bowel disease. Nature. 2011;**474**:307-317. DOI: 10.1038/nature10209

[22] Sifuentes-Dominguez L, Patel AS. Genetics and therapeutics in pediatric ulcerative colitis: The past, present and future. F1000Res. 2016;**5**(F1000 Faculty Rev):240. DOI: 10.12688/f1000research.7440.1

[23] Bousvaros A, Sylvester F, Kugathasan S, Szigethy E, Fiocchi C, et al. Challenges in pediatric inflammatory bowel disease. Inflammatory Bowel Diseases. 2006;**12**:885-913. DOI: 10.1097/01.mib.0000228358.25364.8b

[24] Cuffari C. Diagnostic considerations in pediatric inflammatory bowel disease management. Gastroenterology & Hepatology (NY). 2009;**5**:775-783

[25] Nameirakpam J, Rikhi R, Rawat SS, Sharma J, Suri D. Genetics on early onset inflammatory bowel disease: An update. Genes and Diseases. 2019;**7**:93-106. DOI: 10.1016/j.gendis.2019.10.003

[26] Moran CJ, Klein C, Muise AM, Snapper SB. Very early-onset inflammatory bowel disease: Gaining insight through focused discovery. Inflammatory Bowel Diseases. 2015;**21**:1166-1175. DOI: 10.1097/MIB.0000000000000329

[27] Kugathasan S, Baldassano RN, Bradfield JP, Sleiman PM, Imielinski M, et al. Loci on 20q13 and 21q22 are associated with pediatric-onset inflammatory bowel disease. Nature Genetics. 2008;**40**:1211-1215. DOI: 10.1038/ng.203

[28] Imielinski M, Baldassano RN, Griffiths A, Russell RK, Annese V, et al. Common variants at five new loci associated with early-onset inflammatory bowel disease. Nature Genetics. 2009;**41**:1335-1340. DOI: 10.1038/ng.489

[29] Mamula P, Markowitz JE, Baldassano RN. Inflammatory bowel disease in early childhood and adolescence: Special considerations. Gastroenterology Clinics of North America. 2003;**32**:967-995

[30] Jakobsen C, Bartek J Jr, Wewer V, Vind I, Munkholm P, et al. Differences in phenotype and disease course in adult and paediatric inflammatory bowel disease—a population-based study. Alimentary Pharmacology & Therapeutics. 2011;**34**:1217-1224. DOI: 10.1111/j.1365-2036.2011.04857.x

[31] Jang HJ, Kang B, Choe BH. The difference in extraintestinal manifestations of inflammatory bowel disease for children and adults. Translational Pediatrics. 2019;**8**:4-15. DOI: 10.21037/tp.2019.01.06

[32] Moeeni V, Day AS. Impact of inflammatory bowel disease upon growth in children and adolescents. ISRN Pediatrics. 2011;**2011**:365712. DOI: 10.5402/2011/365712

[33] Ruemmele FM, Turner D. Differences in the management of pediatric and adult-onset ulcerative colitis—lessons from the joint ECCO and ESPGHAN consensus guidelines for the management of pediatric ulcerative colitis. Journal of Crohn's & Colitis. 2014;**8**:1-4. DOI: 10.1016/j.crohns.2013.10.006

[34] Van Limbergen J, Russell RK, Drummond HE, Aldhous MC, Round NK, et al. Definition of phenotypic characteristics of childhood-onset inflammatory bowel disease. Gastroenterology. 2008;**135**:1114-1122. DOI: 10.1053/j.gastro.2008.06.081

[35] Gower-Rousseau C, Dauchet L, Vernier-Massouille G, Tilloy E, Brazier F, et al. The natural history of pediatric ulcerative colitis: A population-based cohort study. The American Journal of Gastroenterology. 2009;**104**:2080-2088. DOI: 10.1038/ajg.2009.177

[36] Malaty HM, Mehta S, Abraham B, Garnett EA, Ferry GD. The natural course of inflammatory bowel disease-indeterminate from childhood to adulthood: Within a 25 year period. Clinical and Experimental Gastroenterology. 2013;**6**:115-121. DOI: 10.2147/CEG.S44700

[37] Abraham BP, Mehta S, El-Serag HB. Natural history of pediatric-onset inflammatory bowel disease: A systematic review. Journal of Clinical Gastroenterology. 2012;**46**:581-589. DOI: 10.1097/MCG.0b013e318247c32f

[38] Rialon KL, Crowley E, Seemann NM, Fahy AS, Muise A, et al. Long-term outcomes for children with very early-onset colitis: Implications for surgical management. Journal of Pediatric Surgery. 2018;**53**:964-967. DOI: 10.1016/j.jpedsurg.2018.02.023

[39] Turner D, Otley AR, Mack D, Hyams J, de Bruijne J, et al. Development,

validation, and evaluation of a pediatric ulcerative colitis activity index: A prospective multicenter study. Gastroenterology. 2007;**133**:423-432. DOI: 10.1053/j.gastro.2007.05.029

[40] Turner D, Ruemmele FM, Orlanski-Meyer E, Griffiths AM, de Carpi JM, et al. Management of paediatric ulcerative colitis, part 1: Ambulatory care-an evidence-based guideline from European Crohn's and Colitis Organization and European Society of Paediatric Gastroenterology, Hepatology and Nutrition. Journal of Pediatric Gastroenterology and Nutrition. 2018;**67**:257-291. DOI: 10.1097/MPG.0000000000002035

[41] Turner D, Ruemmele FM, Orlanski-Meyer E, Griffiths AM, de Carpi JM, et al. Management of paediatric ulcerative colitis, part 2: Acute severe colitis-an evidence-based consensus guideline from the European Crohn's and Colitis Organization and the European Society of Paediatric Gastroenterology, Hepatology and Nutrition. Journal of Pediatric Gastroenterology and Nutrition. 2018;**67**:292-310. DOI: 10.1097/MPG.0000000000002036

[42] Fell JM, Muhammed R, Spray C, Crook K, Russell RK, BSPGHAN IBD working group. Management of ulcerative colitis. Archives of Disease in Childhood. 2016;**101**:469-474. DOI: 10.1136/archdischild-2014-307218

[43] Marshall JK, Thabane M, Steinhart AH, Newman JR, Anand A, et al. Rectal 5-aminosalicylic acid for induction of remission in ulcerative colitis. Cochrane Database of Systematic Reviews. 2010;**20**:CD004115. DOI: 10.1002/14651858.CD004115.pub2

[44] Turner D, Yerushalmi B, Kori M, Broide E, Mozer-Glassberg Y, et al. Once- versus twice-daily mesalazine to induce remission in paediatric ulcerative colitis: A randomised controlled trial. Journal of Crohn's & Colitis. 2017;**11**: 527-533. DOI: 10.1093/ecco-jcc/jjw180

[45] Burri E, Maillard MH, Schoepfer AM, Seibold F, Van Assche G, et al. Treatment algorithm for mild and moderate-to-severe ulcerative colitis: An update. Digestion. 2020;**101**(Suppl. 1):2-15. DOI: 10.1159/000504092

[46] Wilson A, Choi B, Sey M, Ponich T, Beaton M, et al. High infliximab trough concentrations are associated with sustained histologic remission in inflammatory bowel disease: A prospective cohort study. BMC Gastroenterology. 2021;**21**:77. DOI: 10.1186/s12876-021-01650-7

[47] Feuerstein JD, Nguyen GC, Kupfer SS, Falck-Ytter Y, Singh S. American Gastroenterological Association Institute guideline on therapeutic drug monitoring in inflammatory bowel disease. Gastroenterology. 2017;**153**:827-834. DOI: 10.1053/j.gastro.2017.07.032

[48] Papamichael K, Van Stappen T, Vande Casteele N, Gils A, Billiet T, et al. Infliximab concentration thresholds during induction therapy are associated with short-term mucosal healing in patients with ulcerative colitis. Clinical Gastroenterology and Hepatology. 2016;**14**:543-549. DOI: 10.1016/j.cgh.2015.11.014

[49] Lucafò M, Curci D, Bramuzzo M, Alvisi P, Martelossi S, et al. Serum adalimumab levels after induction are associated with long-term remission in children with inflammatory bowel disease. Frontiers in Pediatrics. 2021;**9**:646671. DOI: 10.3389/fped.2021.646671

[50] Turner D, Levine A, Kolho KL, Shaoul R, Ledder O. Combination of oral antibiotics may be effective in severe pediatric ulcerative colitis: A preliminary report. Journal of Crohn's & Colitis. 2014;**8**:1464-1470. DOI: 10.1016/j.crohns.2014.05.010

[51] Turner D, Bishai J, Reshef L, Abitbol G, Focht G, et al. Antibiotic cocktail for pediatric acute severe colitis and the microbiome: The PRASCO randomized controlled trial. Inflammatory Bowel Diseases. 2020;**26**:1733-1742. DOI: 10.1093/ibd/izz298

[52] Müller KE, Lakatos PL, Arató A, Kovács JB, Várkonyi Á, et al. Incidence, Paris classification, and follow-up in a nationwide incident cohort of pediatric patients with inflammatory bowel disease. Journal of Pediatric Gastroenterology and Nutrition. 2013;**57**:576-582. DOI: 10.1097/MPG.0b013e31829f7d8c

[53] Aloi M, D'Arcangelo G, Pofi F, Vassallo F, Rizzo V, et al. Presenting features and disease course of pediatric ulcerative colitis. Journal of Crohn's & Colitis. 2013;**7**:e509-e515. DOI: 10.1016/j.crohns.2013.03.007

[54] Schechter A, Griffiths C, Gana JC, Shaoul R, Shamir R, et al. Early endoscopic, laboratory and clinical predictors of poor disease course in paediatric ulcerative colitis. Gut. 2015;**64**:580-588. DOI: 10.1136/gutjnl-2014-306999

[55] Turner D, Griffiths AM. Acute severe ulcerative colitis in children: A systematic review. Inflammatory Bowel Diseases. 2011;**17**:440-449. DOI: 10.1002/ibd.21383

[56] Barclay AR, Keightley JM, Horrocks I, Garrick V, McGrogan P, et al. Cerebral thromboembolic events in pediatric patients with inflammatory bowel disease. Inflammatory Bowel Diseases. 2010;**16**:677-683. DOI: 10.1002/ibd.21113

[57] Keene DL, Matzinger MA, Jacob PJ, Humphreys P. Cerebral vascular events associated with ulcerative colitis in children. Pediatric Neurology. 2001;**24**:238-243. DOI: 10.1016/s0887-8994(00)00264-2

[58] Nguyen LT, Laberge JM, Guttman FM, Albert D. Spontaneous deep vein thrombosis in childhood and adolescence. Journal of Pediatric Surgery. 1986;**21**:640-643. DOI: 10.1016/s0022-3468(86)80422-5

[59] Benchimol EI, Mack DR, Nguyen GC, Snapper SB, Li W, et al. Incidence, outcomes, and health services burden of very early onset inflammatory bowel disease. Gastroenterology. 2014;**147**:803-813.e7; quiz e14-5. DOI: 10.1053/j.gastro.2014.06.023

[60] Lo B, Zhang K, Lu W, Zheng L, Zhang Q, et al. Autoimmune disease. Patients with LRBA deficiency show CTLA4 loss and immune dysregulation responsive to abatacept therapy. Science. 2015;**349**:436-440. DOI: 10.1126/science.aaa1663

Chapter 7

Ulcerative Colitis and Pregnancy

Athula Kaluarachchi, Nilesh Fernandopulle, Probhodana Ranaweera, Dinindu Kaluarachchi, Indumini Kaluarachchi and Sanupa Kumarasiri Jayawardena

Abstract

Ulcerative colitis (UC) is characterized by relapsing and remitting episodes of inflammation limited to the mucosal layer of the colon. It commonly involves the rectum and may extend to involve other parts of the colon. The age of onset for females is during the reproductive years, and many are likely to get pregnant after the diagnosis of the disease. Women have comparable fertility to the general population when the disease is in remission. Fertility is likely to get affected in women with active disease and in women who had undergone ileal pouch-anal anastomosis (IPAA). Assisted reproduction has improved the chances of successful pregnancy in these women whose fertility is impaired following surgery. Affected females delay pregnancy due to active disease, fear of medications affecting the fetus, and fear of transmitting the disease to the newborn. Most drugs used in the management are safe in pregnancy except for drugs such as methotrexate and tofacitinib. Congenital abnormalities are not increased in pregnancies complicated with ulcerative colitis. Preconception counseling with the objective of planning the pregnancy during remission, reviewing drug therapy, and educating on the importance of continuing medication and its safety are important for better outcomes for the mother and the baby.

Keywords: ulcerative colitis, pregnancy, inflammatory bowel disease, fertility, fetus

1. Introduction

Ulcerative colitis (UC) is an inflammatory bowel disease, sometimes diagnosed during the reproductive years. The incidence and prevalence of ulcerative colitis vary not only according to geographical region but also to race and ethnicity. In an Australian study, the estimated crude prevalence of IBD was 653 per 100,000 patients, Crohn's disease was 306 per 100,000, and ulcerative colitis was 334 per 100,000. In this study, males had a lower risk of Crohn's disease and a higher risk of UC compared to females [1].

In a systematic review and meta-analysis of studies done in the Arab world, quantitative analysis revealed a pooled incidence of 2.33 (95% confidence interval [CI] 1.2–3.4) per 100,000 persons per year for UC and 1.46 (95% CI 1.03–1.89) per 100,000 persons per year for CD [2].

The incidence and prevalence of UC in Latin America were different between regions and studies, ranging from 0.04 to 8.00/100,000 and 0.23 to 76.1/100,000, respectively. An increasing trend was seen over the period from 1986 to 2015. Most patients with UC were females (53.6–72.6%) [3]. In the Asian region, the mean annual incidence of IBD was 1.5 per 100,000. India had the highest incidence of IBD and ulcerative colitis [4].

Approximately 25% of women are likely to get pregnant after the diagnosis of the disease [5]. Prepregnancy counseling and controlling the disease activity before pregnancy are important because active disease at the time of conception and during the pregnancy has shown to result in poor maternal and fetal outcomes [6–9]. Review of drug therapy is also important since some of the drugs such as Methotrexate and Tofacitinib used in the management could affect the fetus.

Active disease during pregnancy is associated with an increased risk of maternal and fetal complications; therefore, it is important to continue therapy and have the disease under control at the time of conception and during pregnancy [6, 7, 9, 10].

Almost 50% of women with IBD have been identified to have a poor knowledge of pregnancy-related issues [11]. Poor knowledge of specific issues related to reproductive health leads to patient concerns and noncompliance. Different educational activities, including eLearning, have shown to improve the patient's knowledge of pregnancy-related issues and reduce patient concerns, which in turn will improve compliance [12, 13]. Current knowledge of prepregnancy assessment of patients with UC, the management of pregnancy, safety and the effects of medication, management of delivery, and the postpartum period will be discussed in this chapter.

2. Prepregnancy planning

Women with UC have a higher risk of adverse pregnancy outcomes than women without the disease. The magnitude of this risk is related to the disease activity at the time of pregnancy. As such, a woman with inflammatory bowel disease needs interventions to manage the disease before pregnancy to minimize adverse outcomes [6, 7, 9, 10]. This is particularly important if the patients have undergone surgical management.

Ulcerative colitis (UC) can affect women during their childbearing years. Pregnancy presents a unique challenge, in the management of UC, where the physician needs to make sure the mother's health is optimally managed, while not compromising the health of the fetus. At most instances, pregnancy in a UC patient would have an uncomplicated course. A multi-disciplinary treatment approach is required when a UC patient becomes pregnant.

2.1 Preconception counseling and education

It is important that patients are advised to conceive during a period of remission of their disease. Prepregnancy planning and proper communication with the treating physician are paramount in this context. Fertility wishes must be discussed with any female with UC in their reproductive age during the consultation and appropriate advice should be given. There are several concerns regarding UC during pregnancy, its impact on pregnancy outcomes, and its effect on the disease. These should be discussed with the patients before pregnancy.

It has been shown that 30–35% of pregnancies are complicated by flares [14]. A meta-analysis of 14 studies found a significantly higher risk ratio of active disease during pregnancy in mothers with UC who commenced pregnancy with active disease (55%) as opposed to the mothers in remission at conception (36%) (risk ratio,

2.0; 95% confidence interval, 1.5–3; P < .001). Similar results were seen in a recent European multicenter cohort: where only 14% of patients in remission at conception relapsed during pregnancy. In contrast, 26% of those with active disease at conception remained in active disease during pregnancy [8].

Having active disease at conception is found to be associated with adverse pregnancy outcomes. In a Danish study of inflammatory bowel disease, 55% of mothers had an inactive disease and 45% had mild to moderate active disease during pregnancy. There was a twofold higher risk of preterm delivery in the active disease group when compared to the disease inactive group [15]. Several such studies have reiterated the importance of the woman being in remission or at least only having mild disease at the time of conception.

When the woman is in remission or has only mild disease activity at the time of conception, it is very likely that the pregnancy will be uncomplicated [16]. A meta-analysis by Miller et al. in more than 1300 female UC patients demonstrated that normal pregnancies are observed in 85% of women with UC (76–97% in individual studies) [17].

In a study by Mountfield et al. on fear and fertility in patients with IBD, 25.8% of patients reported fear of fertility due to ulcerative colitis. This fear was equally seen in males and females suffering from the disease. Only 15.3% have consulted for medical advice before pregnancy in this study. Fear of congenital abnormalities, fear of teratogenicity of drugs, fear of genetic transmission, and inappropriate advice negatively influenced the reproductive decisions. The impact of fertility is variable in different couples as such, it is important to use an individualized approach for prepregnancy advice [18].

Familial occurrence of inflammatory bowel disease (IBD) is well documented. In a study with over 2000 UC patients, a positive family history of IBD was confirmed in 31 patients (1.5%), and 24 (77.4%) had only first-degree relatives affected. All the affected relatives had UC [19]. Different studies have reported varying familial risks of developing ulcerative colitis depending on the study population [20].

The initial prenatal visit is very important to plan out the future pregnancy and communicate and alleviate any concerns of the couple. Discussion should focus on nutritional aspects, weight gain, disease activity, monitoring of mother and fetus, and managing a potential flareup in the future. This discussion that begins at the preconception visit should continue in a dynamic process throughout the pregnancy, further reiterating the importance of management steps.

The principle underlying the treatment of UC during pregnancy is balancing the risks associated with active disease versus any probable or actual risk associated with specific UC medications. Most mothers would feel any medication during pregnancy will be harmful to the baby and would opt not to continue with their medications. It is important this fear is acknowledged and discussed and set into context. Proper counseling of the potential adverse effects of the medications and untreated disease needs to be discussed with the mother and other relevant persons. It is important to communicate with the mother and highlight the importance of continuing the medications and being in remission throughout the pregnancy. Most drugs are considered safe in pregnancy and active disease is likely more harmful than the medication that maintains remission. Medication used by the woman should be reviewed. Medicines which are considered unsafe in pregnancy should be changed to more pregnancy friendly medication when a couple plans a pregnancy. Ideally this should be done at least 3 months prior to the pregnancy, so that there is adequate time for the new medication to take its action and the woman to be in remission at the time of conception.

2.2 Ulcerative colitis and fertility

A systematic review of 11 studies to evaluate nonsurgically treated inflammatory bowel disease found that there is no reduction in fertility in women and men with UC in remission [21]. Lower fertility rates have been reported in women with active disease [22, 23]. However, in UC patients with ileal-pouch anal anastomosis (IPAA), there is an observed reduction in fertility. In a recent meta-analysis, the relative risk of infertility is reported as 4.17 (95% CI 1.99, 8.74) compared with patients before surgery in women who had UC [24]. This is likely due to reproductive organ damage during deep pelvic dissection, formation of scar tissue and adhesions, and the increased prevalence of dyspareunia following surgery.

However, a recent Cochrane review of 16 studies concluded that the effect of surgery on female fertility is uncertain. Any differences in infertility among those undergoing open versus laparoscopic procedures were also uncertain [25].

Assisted reproduction is safe and effective in patients with ulcerative colitis. In medically managed patients, the live birth rates are like that of the general population. However, the live births are reduced after IPAA failure [26].

2.3 Contraception

Since it is advisable to get pregnant during disease remission, contraception plays a significant role in prepregnancy management. Women with UC often present during the reproductive years [5, 7], and thus, women with this disorder need effective contraceptives to prevent unintended pregnancies or to optimally time desired pregnancies.

With regard to oral contraceptives, concerns are expressed about their absorption, increasing the risk of relapses, and increasing the risk of venous thrombosis during their use. In a systematic review on contraceptive use among patients with inflammatory bowel disease, the studies have shown that absorption of the hormones is not affected by the presence of ulcerative colitis, including the patients who had undergone surgery. The frequency or severity of relapses is also not affected compared to nonusers of oral contraceptives. There is no adequate data on the risk of venous thrombosis [27].

Long-term use of depot medroxyprogesterone acetate (DMPA) is associated with small but reversible changes in bone mineral density [28], but it is not known whether the use of DMPA modifies the risk of osteoporosis or osteopenia in women with UC.

Long-acting reversible contraceptives, such as copper or levonorgestrel intrauterine devices or levonorgestrel implants, are highly effective contraceptive methods. Center for Disease Control and Prevention (CDC) recommends the use of these methods for patients with ulcerative colitis [29].

3. Effect of pregnancy on ulcerative colitis activity

Patients with disease remission at the time of conception have 26–35% chance of flare during pregnancy, and this is comparable to the risk of flare in nonpregnant women [7, 8]. There is a significantly higher risk of disease relapse in patients with UC during pregnancy, particularly in the first and second trimesters and the postpartum period compared with nonpregnant women with UC [8, 17]. Similar results were seen in a recent European multicenter cohort: where only 26.4% of patients in remission at conception relapsed during pregnancy. In contrast, 33% of those with active disease at conception remained in active disease until delivery [8]. Most of patients with active disease went into remission during pregnancy [8, 30].

A meta-analysis of 227 women with active UC at conception identified that 24% of women continued to have active disease, 45% experienced worsening disease activity, and 27% improved during pregnancy [17, 30].

In a study with 206 women with IBD, postpartum flares occurred in 31.6% of women, out of which 60% were in patients with UC [31]. The development of postpartum flares was predicted by disease activity during the third trimester, therapy de-escalation during pregnancy, and therapy de-escalation after pregnancy [31].

4. Effect of ulcerative colitis on the pregnancy and child

Many studies have shown that women with UC have an increased risk of preterm delivery, low birth weight (LBW), small-for-gestational-age (SGA), and cesarean section (CS) delivery [30, 32–37]. It has also been shown that these complications are higher in patients with active disease requiring drug therapy [10, 32].

Having active disease at conception is found to be associated with negative pregnancy outcomes as well. In a Danish study of inflammatory bowel disease, 55% of mothers had inactive disease and 45% had mild to moderate active disease during pregnancy. There was a twofold higher risk of preterm delivery in the active disease group when compared to the inactive group [15]. Several such studies have reiterated the importance of the woman being in remission or at least only having mild disease at conception.

If the woman is in remission or has only mild disease activity at conception, it is very likely that the pregnancy will be uncomplicated [16].

Some studies have shown an increased rate of miscarriage in patients with UC compared to the normal population. However, this difference was not statistically significant [38].

Most studies have shown that there is no increased risk of congenital abnormalities in patients with UC compared to patients without the disease [32, 35, 37].

5. Management of a patient with UC during pregnancy

5.1 Obstetrics care

Once pregnant, it is recommended to refer patients with UC for consultant-led care early. An ultrasound scan to exclude an ectopic pregnancy is important, especially in patients who have undergone bowel surgery. After confirming the viability of pregnancy, arranging specialized care in a joint clinic with an experienced obstetrician and IBD physician is recommended for optimal care during pregnancy [39, 40].

Dating the pregnancy with an ultrasound scan between 12 and 14 weeks should be done as there is an increased risk of preterm delivery in a patient with UC. Aneuploidy screening should be performed in line with local guidelines. An anomaly scan to screen for congenital anomalies should be offered to all patients with UC.

Serial growth scans in the third trimester are recommended as there is an increased risk of small for gestational age and fetal growth restriction [30, 32–37].

Vaccinations during pregnancy should be offered as routine, including vaccination against COVID-19, although very limited data is available regarding its safety.

Preliminary studies have shown no significant increased risk with COVID-19 mRNA vaccines during pregnancy [41].

5.2 Nutrition

During pregnancy, the fetus derives all its nutrition from the mother via the placenta. Therefore, the mother's nutrition should be optimal to ensure a healthy baby. IBD patients are at increased risk of macro and micronutrient deficiencies due to mucosal loss and impaired absorption [42]. Zinc, Vitamin D and B12, Calcium, folic acid, iron, and protein deficiencies are known to occur in IBD patients and should be actively suspected and treated as indicated [40, 43, 44].

There are studies that have shown that a diet rich in vegetable oils, fruits, grains, and fish has protective effects on adverse pregnancy outcomes [44].

5.3 Drug therapy and safety during pregnancy

Most medications used in UC are considered safe during pregnancy (**Table 1**). But an honest discussion with the mother is important to ensure compliance.

5.3.1 5 Aminosalicylates (5 ASA)

Aminosalicylates are used in the treatment of mild to moderate UC. Aminosalicylates are generally considered safe for use in pregnancy as per the European Crohn's and colitis guidelines (ECCO) [45]. Several case series, population-based cohort studies, and two meta-analyses did not demonstrate an increased risk for early pregnancy adverse outcomes such as miscarriage and ectopic pregnancy in mothers continuing with 5 ASA during pregnancy [46]. Few trials have demonstrated premature birth and low birth weight with 5 ASA use, but whether active disease during pregnancy was considered a confounding factor cannot be ascertained [46]. Reassuringly, animal and human data, including recent meta-analysis, did not demonstrate any teratogenic effects with 5 ASA and therefore is recommended to be continued during pregnancy [47]. Sulfasalazine can potentially interfere with folate

Medication	Risk during pregnancy	FDA category
Mesalazine	Low risk	B
Sulphasalazine	Low risk	B
Corticosteroids	Low risk	C
Thiopurines	Low risk (Limited data for 6 TG)	D
Anti TNF Agents	Low risk, consider stopping in 3rd trimester if in remission	B
Methotrexate	Do not take during pregnancy	X
Metronidazole	Avoid in the first trimester	B
Ciprofloxacin	Avoid in the first trimester	C
Tofacitinib	No reliable human studies are available	C

Table 1.
Summary of medications used in ulcerative colitis.

absorption, which is essential for neural tube development. Folic acid supplementation is therefore always required if not already given.

5.3.2 Corticosteroids

Steroids are needed in the management of most acute flares of UC and are recommended for use in the ECCO guidelines [45]. Corticosteroid may increase the risk of pregnancy-related adverse outcomes and gestational diabetes. Although most studies have not shown an increased risk of congenital malformations associated with the use of steroids, there seems to be an increased risk of orofacial malformations if steroids are used in the first trimester [48]. However, a large population-based study, including 51,973 pregnancies, did not show any adverse events from using steroids during pregnancy [49].

5.3.3 Ciclosporin and tacrolimus

Both ciclosporin and tacrolimus are widely used for the treatment of solid organ transplantation, and most data on pregnancy outcomes are derived from such patients. In a meta-analysis of 15 studies with 410 pregnant patients, ciclosporin did not cause an increased rate of congenital malformations [50]. Data on pregnant women with IBD are minimal.

5.3.4 Thiopurine

Thiopurines, both azathioprine and 6-mercaptopurine, are used in the maintenance of remission of UC and are considered low risk and well tolerated during pregnancy [45].

Thiopurine use in pregnancy has been evaluated in several studies. Initial studies showed an increased risk of preterm delivery, small for gestational age and low birth weight, [51, 52] but these studies overall failed to consider disease activity, which is commonly associated with these pregnancy outcomes. On the contrary, several recent studies revealed thiopurines did not cause any negative pregnancy outcomes [53, 54]. With respect to congenital anomalies, studies have revealed an association with thiopurine use in pregnancy, but again several long-term studies have refuted these findings, adding up to the debate on the safety of thiopurines in pregnancy [55–57]. In a Spanish study, interestingly, patients on thiopurines had better pregnancy-related outcomes than those not exposed to thiopurines, further emphasizing the importance of controlling the disease throughout pregnancy [53, 58].

5.3.5 Biologics

Although there is substantial evidence of its safety in pregnancy, some mothers may insist on stopping biologics during pregnancy. Discontinuation of biological therapy early during pregnancy poses several problems. There is a potential risk of flares during pregnancy and postpartum period, increased risk of developing antibodies against the biologics, and possible loss of response if restarting is needed. Therefore, discontinuation of biologics during pregnancy should only be considered under certain circumstances in patients who are at a very low risk of relapse. Studies have shown patients may be considered low risk if objective sustained endoscopic remission is seen for 6 months before conception, appropriate therapeutic levels before conception, no hospitalization in the last 3 years, no prior bowel resection, no previous loss of response to anti-TNFs, or need for dose optimization [59].

5.3.5.1 Anti-TNF agents

Anti-TNF agents used for IBD include infliximab (IFX), adalimumab, golimumab, and in some countries certolizumab (CZP). Anti-TNF agents do not cross the placenta passively as they are large molecules. However, as their structure resembles maternal immunoglobulins that are transported actively from the end of the second trimester, they too can be actively transported across the placenta. Therefore, not only is the fetus potentially exposed to these agents, but they can have blood levels exceeding maternal levels [60]. In contrast to the other anti-TNF agents, certolizumab has a pegylated molecular structure and is not transferred across or has very low or no detectable fetal drug levels at birth [61]. As organogenesis occurs before this transplacental anti-TNF drug transfer, there are no reported congenital malformations with the use of biological agents. In the PIANO (Pregnancy Inflammatory bowel disease And Neonatal Outcomes) registry, more than 500 women were exposed to the anti-TNF medications during pregnancy, and no increased risk of adverse pregnancy outcomes was reported [62]. Several studies have shown anti-TNF agents do not increase pregnancy-related outcomes [53, 63] and are therefore considered low risk and recommended for being used in pregnancy in the ECCO guidelines [45]. It is important to delay the scheduled dose of anti-TNF agents as late as possible during the second trimester (around 24–26 weeks of gestation), to maintain remission during the third trimester and to limit its transport to the fetus [64].

Infliximab has been detected at 6 months after birth in the child; therefore, there have been concerns about its implications on neonatal vaccinations. No adverse outcomes have been reported for non-live vaccines [65]. It s recommended to only institute live vaccines after 6 months of age when no detectable anti-TNF medication is seen in the child's blood. Levels of other immune suppressants used in pregnancy are probably not elevated in neonates, and routine vaccination schedules can be followed, although reliable data are lacking.

5.3.5.2 Anti-integrin agents – Vedolizumab

Vedolizumab (VDZ) is unique as it is a gut-selective IgG-1 monoclonal antibody against the integrin $\alpha4\beta7$. There is limited data on the effects of VDZ in pregnancy. A small case series consisting of 24 and 73 pregnancies exposed to VDZ had no safety concerns reported [66, 67].

In a European retrospective study, no difference in miscarriages was seen with VDZ exposed and a control group on IFX (16 vs. 13%, $p = 0.71$) or a control group not exposed to any biologics (16 vs. 10%, $p = 0.236$). Similar number of miscarriages were seen once patients with active disease were excluded from the analysis [68]. It is recommended to use VDZ in pregnancy if indicated. But, if the childbearing age woman is naïve to biologics, as most data are available with anti-TNF agents, anti-TNFs, especially CZP, are most appropriate as a first-line treatment option for use of biologics in pregnancy.

5.3.5.3 Ustekinumab

Ustekinumab is increasingly used in pregnancy, and like the other anti-TNF agents, it is an actively transported IgG1 antibody across the placenta via neonatal Fc receptors. It appears to have stable drug levels during pregnancy, with a similar infant: maternal ratio of the older anti-TNFs. It is completely cleared from the infant's blood by 20 weeks. But like with other biologics, live vaccination needs to be avoided at least till 12 months of age until further clearance data are obtained [69].

5.3.5.4 Tofacitinib

Animal studies clearly show congenital malformations with tofacitinib in supra therapeutic doses. Although no reliable human studies are available, it is recommended to avoid this drug, especially in the first trimester. As the half-life of the drug is short, a washout period of approximately 1 week is adequate before conception [67].

5.4 Disease assessment and monitoring of UC

As IBD may adversely affect pregnancy and vice versa, it is important that the activity of the disease is objectively monitored before pregnancy and during a flair within the duration of the pregnancy. Various modalities are used to assess disease activity in IBD.

Along with histology, direct visualization with endoscopy is the definitive method to assess disease activity in IBD. But procedure-related hazards to the mother and fetus, including fetal hypoxia and demise, maternal positioning for the endoscopy and maternal hypotension, and sedation during pregnancy, are a concern [70].

Due to physiological changes in pregnancy haeamoglobin, albumin are lower and erythrocyte sedimentation rate (ESR) is higher than normal, therefore these should not be used to monitor disease activity. Fecal calprotectin that measures gastrointestinal mucosal inflammation is detected before clinical symptoms and is a useful noninvasive indicator of disease activity, although its use specifically in pregnancy has not been studied. Fecal calprotectin of lower than 50 ug/g has been shown to be predictive of quiescent disease in UC [71].

5.5 Management of flare and acute severe ulcerative colitis in pregnancy

Management of flares in UC would be like a nonpregnant patient. Serum biomarkers used traditionally to assess severity of UC may be physiologically abnormal during pregnancy.

Steroid therapy: The steroid regime is IV methylprednisolone 40 mg BD or IV hydrocortisone 100 mg QDS and rectal Hydrocortisone 100 mg in 100 ml normal saline BD given through soft rectal cannula (Foley catheter) over 30 minutes, via IV giving set.

Dehydration: Administer IV fluids to correct dehydration, with at least 60 mmol potassium per day. Patients are highly prone to hypokalemia due to diarrhea and steroid therapy, and this requires close attention.

Anti-coagulation: Prophylactic doses of LMW heparin should be considered in all pregnant females with acute relapse, as pregnancy and acute severe UC greatly predisposes a patient to venous thrombosis.

Antibiotics: Metronidazole and ciprofloxacin can be considered for patients suspected of infection after recent hospital admission, visit to an endemic area for amoebiasis, the first attack of UC, or when surgery is considered. In the absence of these features and especially in pregnancy, antibiotics are not routinely indicated [72].

Rescue therapy: Both infliximab and cyclosporine are equally effective and can be considered as rescue therapy in patients who do not respond to first-line therapy.

5.6 Endoscopy during pregnancy

Endoscopy during pregnancy is considered safe if indicated, except in states of placental abruption, ruptured membranes, or eclampsia. It should be performed by an experienced endoscopist and, if possible, should be postponed until after the first trimester. While performing the lower gastrointestinal endoscopy, mothers need to be lying in a left lateral position or what is known as "left pelvic tilt" to avoid compression to the major vessels supplying the placenta. Unsedated flexible sigmoidoscopy is preferred following an enema and would give the necessary information in a patient with UC [73].

If strongly indicated, colonoscopy can be done with obstetric anesthesia monitoring, but colonoscopy is generally avoided due to the difficulties in bowel preparation, technical difficulties, and negative effects on pregnancy. Sedation needs to be discussed with anesthetists, and benzodiazepines are best avoided during pregnancy. It is recommended to document the fetal heartbeat before and after endoscopy and to always have obstetric support available.

5.7 Timing, planning, and management of the delivery of the fetus

In the majority of patients with UC, the mode and timing of delivery can be decided according to the obstetric indications. There is no contraindication for vaginal delivery in a patient with UC without fetal or maternal complications. Episiotomy should be given, if necessary. Vacuum or forceps deliveries should be done for usual obstetrics indications.

When deciding the mode of delivery, the AGA guideline would be a good reference (**Figure 1**) [40]. Patients without perineal disease should be encouraged for vaginal delivery. However, for patients with active disease or with perineal disease (anorectal fistula, anal abscess, rectovaginal fistula, anal fissures, and anal stenosis), cesarean

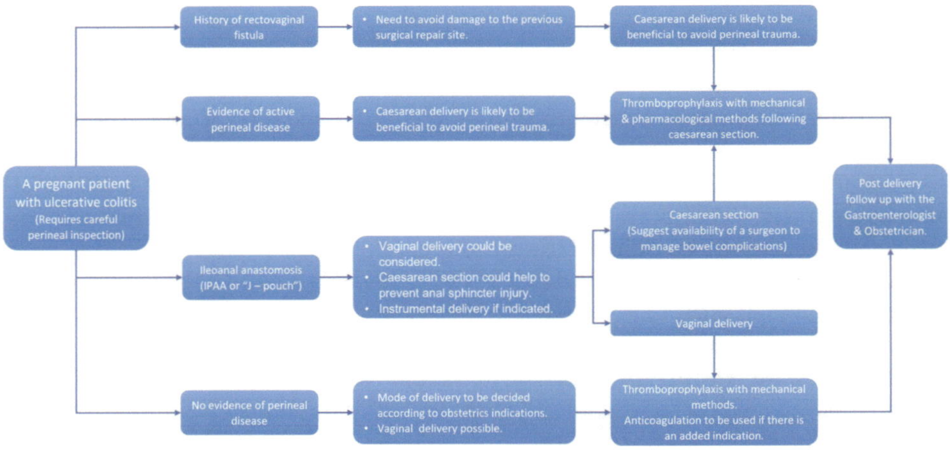

Figure 1.
Guide to decide the mode of delivery in patients with UC. VTE, venous thromboembolism.

delivery should be offered [74]. IPAA is a relative contraindication for vaginal delivery. One should consider the possible protection of anal sphincter by performing an elective cesarean delivery. An experienced obstetrician should perform the cesarean section to minimize the risk of intraoperative organ injury with the possible involvement of the surgical team if required.

Nevertheless, women with UC have a higher risk of cesarean deliveries compared to women in the general population [75]. Most of the time, a cesarean section is suggested or requested because of unjustified fears on the part of patients or care providers.

6. Breast feeding, postpartum management, and follow up including family planning

6.1 Thromboprophylaxis

Patients with UC have an increased risk of developing venous thromboembolism (VTE), especially during the postpartum period [76]. The need for thromboprophylaxis should be assessed in each patient according to AGA guideline [40] (**Figure 1**). Thromboembolic deterrent stockings and low molecular weight heparin (LMWH) should be offered to all women who have undergone cesarean delivery. UC patients with other risk factors for VTE regardless of the mode of delivery should be offered with both mechanical and LMWH as thromboprophylaxis. Some may need anticoagulation for an extended period. LMWH and warfarin can be used in these circumstances. UC patients who have been successful in vaginal delivery with no other risk factors for VTE can be offered mechanical thromboprophylaxis only.

6.2 Postpartum

The risk of relapse is higher during the postpartum period. Discontinuation of drug therapy during pregnancy and fear of drug therapy during breastfeeding are the main reasons. In one study, 75% of cases experienced a relapse during the postpartum period in patients who discontinued the drug treatment before 30 weeks of gestation. In contrast, only 26% of cases had a relapse in patients who continued the drug therapy throughout pregnancy [77].

Biological treatment can be restarted 24 hours after vaginal delivery and 48 hours after cesarean delivery [78]. However, exclusion of possible infection is mandatory before recommencing treatment. Methotrexate can be restarted during the postpartum period if the mother is not breastfeeding [79]. Most of the other drug therapies can be safely continued in the postpartum period (**Figure 2**).

Patients with IPAA are at a higher risk of developing paralytic ileus during the postpartum period, especially the ones who undergo cesarean deliveries. Early feeding and mobilization, proper hydration, and other supportive measures can reduce this risk significantly [80].

The risk of stoma complications is higher during the postpartum period. Liaising with a stoma specialist nurse and colorectal surgeon will help to minimize complications with stoma [79]. Covering the ostomy with a gauze towel is recommended to protect the operative field during cesarean section [76].

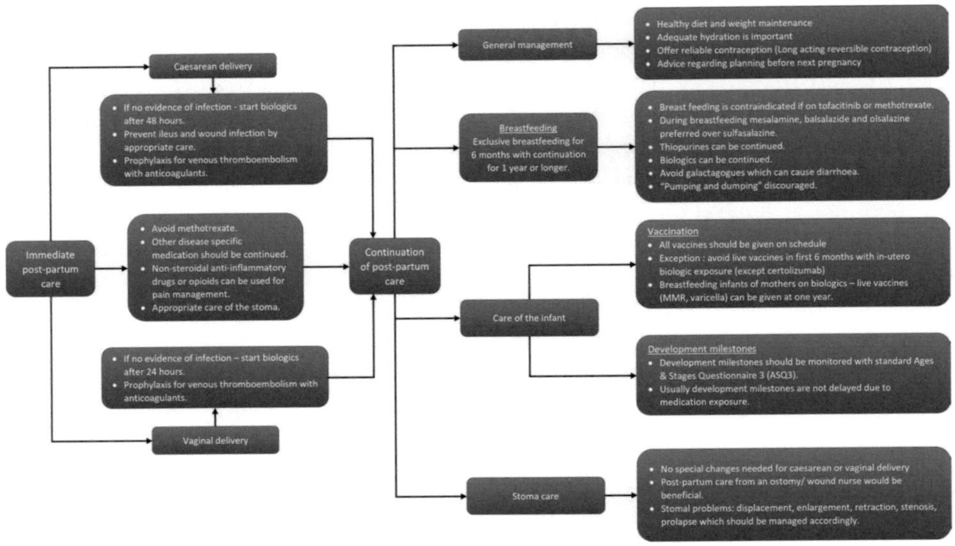

Figure 2.
Postpartum care for women with UC.

6.3 Lactation

In most instances, a woman with UC can breastfeed the child without any major issues. Exclusive breastfeeding for 6 months, with the continuation of breastfeeding for 1 year or longer as mutually desired by mother and infant is recommended. However, a significant number of women with UC defer breastfeeding due to fear of drugs in breast milk or discontinuing medication during the postpartum period, equally harmful to both the mother and baby. In the PIANO registry, the breastfeeding rate was significantly lower in women on immunomodulators and biologic treatments [81].

Breastfeeding has a protective effect on the development of UC in offspring. A systematic review has shown that ever being breastfed was associated with a lower risk of UC (OR 0.78, 95% CI 0.67–0.91) [82].

When deciding the drug therapy during the postpartum period and lactation, the AGA guideline will be very helpful [40].

5-ASA agents (mesalamine, basaloid, and olsalazine) can be continued when breastfeeding. Although they are excreted in breastmilk, only a few isolated cases of diarrhea are reported in infants who are exposed. Compared to sulfasalazine, which is excreted into milk and known to have hemolytic and antimicrobial properties, mesalamine derivatives are safer during lactation [83].

Thiopurines and corticosteroids are secreted in minute amounts in breast milk. Some studies have shown when corticosteroid dose is higher than 20 mg per day, significant levels are detected in breast milk [84]. They can also reduce breast milk production. Some advice avoiding breastfeeding for 3 to 4 hours after taking thiopurines as the drug is not detected in breast milk after 4 hours of dosing. Most of the biological agents are found in minute amounts in breast milk and are degraded in the stomach of the infant, and no significant adverse effects are reported, thus can continue during breastfeeding [85].

Anti-interleukin 12–23 and anti-integrin are considered safe during lactation, as only minute amount is secreted in breastmilk. Nevertheless, limited safety data are available for these relatively new therapies [86].

Due to lack of data, lactation is contraindicated in women who are on tofacitinib.

6.4 Postpartum contraception

Effective, safe, and reliable contraception should be offered to all women with UC after delivery. Long-acting reversible contraceptives are the safest and most effective. These include hormonal or nonhormonal intrauterine devices or hormonal implants. Estrogen-containing contraceptive methods may increase the risk of venous thromboembolism, hence should be offered only if no personnel or family history of DVT or no other risk factors. Estrogen patches or low-dose estrogen contraceptive pills are safer.

7. Long-term effects of ulcerative colitis on the Fetus

7.1 Ulcerative colitis and genetics

Genetic studies have shown an increased risk of developing UC in the offspring, although the risk is somewhat less than Crohn's disease. Family history with multiple members having the disease increases the risk further for the offspring. In monozygotic twins, there is a 6–19% concordance for UC [87]. The incidence rate ratio is 3.7 for UC in an offspring if the mother is having UC and the absolute risk of an offspring developing UC is 1.6% [88]. The risk of developing IBD rises to 30% if both parents have UC [89]. There are no genetic tests available currently to predict the probability of a child developing the disease.

7.2 Infection and vaccination

There is a significant risk of neonatal infection postdelivery due to immunosuppressive treatment during pregnancy. Neonates and infants should be monitored for possible infections, especially if they are exposed to a combination of thiopurines and biologics [79].

It is recommended to avoid live vaccinations until 6 months postdelivery in infants exposed to biological therapy during the third trimester [39]. This is because of possible immunosuppression in the infant due to clinically significant drug levels detected up to 6 months after birth.

7.3 Mental development

PIANO registry data and other studies indicate that there is no significant effect on the neurodevelopment of babies regardless of exposure to the antenatal medication. In fact, some studies have shown better achievement of neurodevelopment milestones in infants with higher drug levels compared to infants with lower drug levels at birth. Therefore, good disease control with proper medication should be encouraged when counseling women with UC [90].

8. Conclusion

Ulcerative colitis affects women during their reproductive years and many of them are likely to plan pregnancy after the diagnosis of the disease. Fertility is reduced in women with active disease and in patients who have undergone surgical management.

Development of advanced fertility management has improved the chances of pregnancy in these women. Prepregnancy assessment of the disease activity, counseling regarding the fetal and maternal outcome, and safety and importance of continuation of medication are important aspects of management of patients affected by ulcerative colitis. Because the pregnancy outcome is adversely affected by disease activity, adequate attention should be given to the continuation of treatment during pregnancy. Most of the drugs used in the management of ulcerative colitis are safe in pregnancy with a few exceptions. Multidisciplinary team management, including gastroenterologist, obstetrician, and neonatologist will help to reduce complications and improve maternal and neonatal outcomes.

Conflict of interest

The authors declare no conflict of interest.

Author details

Athula Kaluarachchi[1*], Nilesh Fernandopulle[1], Probhodana Ranaweera[1], Dinindu Kaluarachchi[2], Indumini Kaluarachchi[3] and Sanupa Kumarasiri Jayawardena[4]

1 Faculty of Medicine, University of Colombo, Sri Lanka

2 Colombo North Teaching Hospital, Ragama, Sri Lanka

3 Faculty of Medical Sciences, University of Sri Jayewardenepura, Sri Lanka

4 Colombo South Teaching Hospital, Kalubowila, Sri Lanka

*Address all correspondence to: athula.kal@gmail.com

References

[1] Busingye D, Pollack A, Chidwick K. Prevalence of inflammatory bowel disease in the Australian general practice population: A cross-sectional study. PLoS One. 2021;**16**(5):e0252458

[2] Mosli M, Alawadhi S, Hasan F, Abou Rached A, Sanai F, Danese S. Incidence, prevalence, and clinical epidemiology of inflammatory bowel disease in the Arab world: A systematic review and Meta-analysis. Inflammation and Intestinal Diseases. 2021;**6**(3):123-131

[3] Kotze PG, Steinwurz F, Francisconi C, Zaltman C, Pinheiro M, Salese L, et al. Review of the epidemiology and burden of ulcerative colitis in Latin America. Therapeutic Advanced Gastroenterology. 2020;**13**:175

[4] Ng SC, Kaplan GG, Tang W, Banerjee R, Adigopula B, Underwood FE, et al. Population density and risk of inflammatory bowel disease: A prospective population-based study in 13 countries or regions in Asia-Pacific. The American Journal of Gastroenterology. 2019;**114**(1):107-115. DOI: 10.1038/s41395-018-0233-2

[5] Ng SC, Shi HY, Hamidi N, Underwood FE, Tang W, Benchimol EI, et al. Worldwide incidence, and prevalence of inflammatory bowel disease in the 21st century: A systematic review of population-based studies. Lancet. 2018;**390**(10114):2769-2778

[6] Abhyankar A, Ham M, Moss AC. Meta-analysis: The impact of disease activity at conception on disease activity during pregnancy in patients with inflammatory bowel disease. Alimentary Pharmacology & Therapeutics. 2013;**38**(5):460-466

[7] Pedersen N, Bortoli A, Duricova D, Inca R, Panelli MR, Gisbert JP, et al. The course of inflammatory bowel disease during pregnancy and postpartum: A prospective European ECCO-EpiCom Study of 209 pregnant women. Alimentary Pharmacology & Therapeutics. 2013;**38**(5):501-512

[8] Bortoli A, Pedersen N, Duricova D, et al. Pregnancy outcome in inflammatory bowel disease: Prospective European case-control ECCO-EpiCom study, 2003-2006. Alimentary Pharmacology & Therapeutics. 2011;**34**:724-734

[9] Bröms G, Granath F, Linder M, Stephansson O, Elmberg M, Kieler H. Birth outcomes in women with inflammatory bowel disease: Effects of disease activity and drug exposure. Inflammatory Bowel Diseases. 2014;**20**(6):1091-1098

[10] Getahun D, Fassett M, Longstreth G, et al. Association between maternal inflammatory bowel disease and adverse perinatal outcomes. Journal of Perinatology. 2014;**34**:435-440

[11] Selinger CP, Eaden J, Selby W, Jones DB, Katelaris P, Chapman G, et al. Patients' knowledge of pregnancy-related issues in inflammatory bowel disease and validation of a novel assessment tool ('CCPKnow'). Alimentary Pharmacology & Therapeutics. 2012;**36**(1):57-63

[12] Reed T, Wierstra K, et al. Pregnancy-related beliefs and concerns of inflammatory bowel disease patients modified after accessing e-health portal. Journal of the Canadian Association of Gastroenterology. 2021;**4**(1):27-35

[13] Williams AJ, Karimi N, Chari R, et al. Shared decision making in pregnancy in inflammatory bowel disease: Design of a patient orientated decision aid. BMC Gastroenterology. 2021;**21**:302

[14] Caprilli R, Gassull MA, Escher JC, et al. European evidence-based consensus on the diagnosis and management of Crohn's disease: Special situations. Gut. 2006;**55**(Suppl. 1):i36-i58

[15] Norgard B, Hundborg HH, Jacobsen BA, et al. Disease activity in pregnant women with Crohn's disease and birth outcomes: A regional Danish cohort study. The American Journal of Gastroenterology. 2007;**102**:1947-1954

[16] Hanan IM. Inflammatory bowel disease in the pregnant woman. Comprising Therapy. 1998;**24**:409-414

[17] Miller JP. Inflammatory bowel-disease in pregnancy a review. Journal of Royal Society of Medicine. 1986;**79**:221-225

[18] Mountifield R, Bampton P, Prosser R, et al. Fear and fertility in inflammatory bowel disease: A mismatch of perception and reality affects family planning decisions. Inflammatory Bowel Diseases. 2009;**15**:720-725

[19] Gupta A, Bopanna S, Kedia S, Yadav DP, Goyal S, Jain S, et al. Familial aggregation of inflammatory bowel disease in patients with ulcerative colitis. Intestinal Research. 2017;**15**:388-394

[20] Santos MPC, Gomes C, Torres J. Familial and ethnic risk in inflammatory bowel disease. Annals of Gastroenterology. 2018;**31**:14-23

[21] Tavernier N, Fumery M, Peyrin-Biroulet L, Colombel JF, Gower-Rousseau C. Systematic review: Fertility in non-surgically treated inflammatory bowel disease. Alimentary Pharmacology & Therapeutics. 2013;**38**(8):847-853

[22] Oresland T, Palmblad S, Ellstrom M, Berndtsson I, Crona N, Hulte´ n L. Gynaecological and sexual function related to anatomical changes in the female pelvis after restorative proctocolectomy. International Journal of Colorectal Diseases. 1994;**9**:77-81

[23] New-Olsen K, Joelsson M, Laurberg S, Oresland T. Fertility after ileal pouch-anal anastomosis in women with ulcerative colitis. The British Journal of Surgery. 1999;**86**:493-495

[24] Sriranganathan D, Poo S, Segal JP. The impact of the ileoanal pouch on female fertility in ulcerative colitis: A systematic review and meta-analysis. Colorectal Disease. Aug 2022;**24**(8):918-924. DOI: 10.1111/codi.16123. Epub 2022 Apr 8. PMID: 35322933

[25] Lee S, Crowe M, Seow CH, et al. The impact of surgical therapies for inflammatory bowel disease on female fertility. Cochrane Database System Review. 2019;**7**:CD012711

[26] Laube R, Tran Y, Paramsothy S, Leong RW. Assisted reproductive technology in Crohn's disease and ulcerative colitis: A Systematic review and meta-analysis. The American Journal of Gastroenterology. 2021;**116**:2334

[27] Lauren B et al. Contraceptive use among women with inflammatory bowel disease: A systematic review. Contraception. 2010;**82**(1):72-85

[28] Curtis KM, Martins S. Progestogen-only contraception and bone mineral density: A systematic review. Contraception. 2006;**73**:470-487

[29] Division of Reproductive Health, National Center for Chronic Disease Prevention and Health Promotion. US Medical Eligibility Criteria (US MEC) for Contraceptive Use. 2016. Retrieved from https://www.cdc.gov/reproductivehealth/contraception/mmwr/mec/summary.html

[30] Laube R, Paramsothy S, Leong RW. Review of pregnancy in Crohn's disease and ulcerative colitis. Therapeutic Advances in Gastroenterology. 18 May 2021;**14**:17562848211016242. DOI: 10.1177/17562848211016242. PMID: 34046084; PMCID: PMC8135214

[31] Yu A, Friedman S, Ananthakrishnan AN. Incidence and predictors of flares in the postpartum year among women with inflammatory bowel disease. Inflammatory Bowel Diseases. 2020;**26**(12):1926-1932

[32] Stephansson O, Larsson H, Pedersen L, Kieler H, Granath F, Ludvigsson JF, et al. Congenital abnormalities and other birth outcomes in children born to women with ulcerative colitis in Denmark and Sweden. Inflammatory Bowel Diseases. 2011;**17**(3):795-801

[33] Herng-Ching L et al. Ulcerative colitis and pregnancy outcomes in an Asian population. American Journal of Gastroenterology. 2010;**105**:387-394

[34] Bengtson MB, Solberg IC, Aamodt G, et al. Relationships between inflammatory bowel disease and perinatal factors: Both maternal and paternal disease are related to preterm birth of offspring. Inflammatory Bowel Diseases. 2010;**16**:847-855

[35] Kammerlander H, Nielsen J, Kjeldsen J, Knudsen T, Friedman S, Nørgård B. The effect of disease activity on birth outcomes in a Nationwide cohort of women with moderate to severe inflammatory bowel disease. Inflammatory Bowel Diseases. 2017;**23**(6):1011-1018

[36] Shand AW, Chen JS, Selby W, Solomon M, Roberts CL. Inflammatory bowel disease in pregnancy: A population-based study of prevalence and pregnancy outcomes. BJOG : An International Journal of Obstetrics and Gynaecology. 2016;**123**(11):1862-1870

[37] Restellini S, Biedermann L, Hruz P, Mottet C, Moens A, Ferrante M, et al. Update on the Management of Inflammatory Bowel Disease during Pregnancy and Breastfeeding. Digestion. 2020;**101**(1):27-42

[38] Lee HH, Bae JM, Lee BI, Lee KM, Wie JH, Kim JS, et al. Pregnancy outcomes in women with inflammatory bowel disease: A 10-year nationwide population-based cohort study. Alimentary Pharmacology & Therapeutics. 2020;**51**(9):861-869

[39] Selinger C, Carey N, Cassere S, et al. Standards for the provision of antenatal care for patients with inflammatory bowel disease: Guidance endorsed by the British Society of Gastroenterology and the British maternal and Fetal medicine society frontline. Gastroenterology. 2021;**12**:182-187

[40] Mahadevan U, Robinson C, Bernasko N, Boland B, Chambers C, Dubinsky M, et al. Inflammatory bowel disease in pregnancy clinical care pathway: A report from the American Gastroenterological Association IBD parenthood project working group. Gastroenterology. 2019;**156**(5):1508-1524

[41] Shimabukuro TT, Kim SY, Myers TR, Moro PL, Oduyebo T, et al. Preliminary findings of mRNA Covid-19 vaccine safety in pregnant persons. New England Journal of Medicine. 2021;**384**:2273-2282

[42] Barker DJP, Clark PM. Fetal undernutrition and disease in later life. Reviews of Reproduction. 1997;**2**:105-112

[43] Goh J, O'Morain CA. Review article: Nutrition and adult inflammatory bowel disease. Alimentary Pharmacology & Therapeutics. 2003;**17**:307-320

[44] Englund-Ögge L, Brantsæter AL, Sengpiel V, et al. Maternal dietary patterns and preterm delivery: Results from large prospective cohort study. BMJ. 2014;**348**:g1446

[45] van der Woude CJ, Ardizzone S, Bengtson MB, Fiorino G, Fraser G, Katsanos K, et al. The second European evidenced-based consensus on reproduction and pregnancy in inflammatory bowel disease. Journal of Crohns Colitis. 2015;**9**(2):107-124

[46] Norgard B, Fonager K, Pedersen L, Jacobsen BA, Sorensen HT. Birth outcome in women exposed to 5-aminosalicylic acid during pregnancy: A Danish cohort study. Gut. 2003;**52**:243-247

[47] Rahimi R, Nikfar S, Rezaie A, Abdollahi M. Pregnancy outcome in women with inflammatory bowel disease following exposure to 5-aminosalicylic acid drugs: A meta-analysis. Reproduction in Toxicology. 2008;**25**:271-275

[48] Park-Wyllie L, Mazzotta P, Pastuszak A, Moretti ME, Beique L, Hunnisett L, et al. Birth defects after maternal exposure to corticosteroids: Prospective cohort study and meta-analysis of epidemiological studies. Teratology. 2000;**62**(6):385-392

[49] Gur C, Diav-Citrin O, Shechtman S, Arnon J, Ornoy A. Pregnancy outcome after first trimester exposure to corticosteroids: A prospective controlled study. Reproductive Toxicology. 2004;**18**(1):93-101

[50] Bar-Oz B, Hackman R, Einarson T, Koren G. Pregnancy outcome after cyclosporine therapy during pregnancy: A meta-analysis. Transplantation. 2001;**71**:1051-1055

[51] Akbari M, Shah S, Velayos FS, Mahadevan U, Cheifetz AS. Systematic review and meta-analysis on the effects of thiopurines on birth outcomes from female and male patients with inflammatory bowel disease. Inflammation Bowel Diseases. 2013;**19**:15-22

[52] Dotan I, Alper A, Rachmilewitz D, et al. Maternal inflammatory bowel disease has short and long-term effects on the health of their offspring: A multicenter study in Israel. Journal of Crohns Colitis. 2013;**7**:542-550

[53] Casanova MJ, Chaparro M, Domènech E, Barreiro-de Acosta M, Bermejo F, Iglesias E, et al. Safety of thiopurines and anti-TNF-α drugs during pregnancy in patients with inflammatory bowel disease. The American Journal of Gastroenterology. 2013;**108**(3):433-440

[54] Molnar T, Farkas K, Nagy F, et al. Pregnancy outcome in patients with inflammatory bowel disease according to the activity of the disease and the medical treatment: A case-control study. Scandinavian Journal of Gastroenterology. 2010;**45**:1302-1306

[55] Ng SW, Mahadevan U. Management of inflammatory bowel disease in pregnancy. Experiment Review in Clinical Immunology. 2013;**9**:161-174

[56] Kanis SL, de Lima-Karagiannis A, BoerNKH D, et al. Use of thiopurines during conception and pregnancy is not associated with adverse pregnancy outcomes or health of infants at one year in a prospective study. Clinical Gastroenterology and Hepatology. 2017;**15**:1232-1241

[57] Goldstein LH, Dolinsky G, Greenberg R, et al. Pregnancy outcome of women exposed to azathioprine during pregnancy. Birth Defects Research Part A. Clinical Molecular in Teratology. 2007;**79**:696-701

[58] Mahadevan U, Dubinsky MC, Su C, Lawendy N, Jones TV, Marren A, et al. Outcomes of pregnancies with maternal/paternal exposure in the tofacitinib safety databases for ulcerative colitis. Inflammatory Bowel Diseases. 2018;**24**(12):2494-2500

[59] Torres J, Boyapati RK, Kennedy NA, Louis E, Colombel JF, Satsangi J. Systematic review of effects of withdrawal of immunomodulators or biologic agents from patients with inflammatory bowel disease. Gastroenterology. 2015;**149**(7):1716-1730

[60] Julsgaard M, Christensen LA, Gibson PR, Gearry RB, Fallingborg J, Hvas CL, et al. Concentrations of adalimumab and infliximab in mothers and Newborns, and effects on infection. Gastroenterology. 2016;**151**(1):110-119

[61] Mahadevan U, Wolf DC, Dubinsky M, et al. Placental transfer of anti-tumor necrosis factor agents in pregnant patients with inflammatory bowel disease. Clinical Gastroenterology and Hepatology. 2013;**11**(3):286-292

[62] Mahadevan U, Martin C, Sandler R, Kane SV, Dubinsky M, Lewis JD, et al. PIANO: A 1000 patient prospective registry of pregnancy outcomes in women with IBD exposed to immunomodulators and biologic therapy [abstract]. Gastroenterology. 2012;**142**(5):142

[63] Flanagan E, Gibson PR, Wright EK, et al. Infliximab, adalimumab and vedolizumab concentrations across pregnancy and vedolizumab concentrations in infants following intrauterine exposure. Alimentary Pharmacology & Therapeutics. 2020;**52**(10):1551-1562

[64] Djokanovic N, Klieger-Grossmann C, Pupco A, Koren G. Safety of infliximab use during pregnancy. Reproduction in Toxicology. 2011;**32**:93-97

[65] Mahadevan U. Pregnancy and inflammatory bowel disease. Gastroenterology in Clinical North America. 2013;**38**:1097-1098

[66] Mahadevan U, Vermeire S, Lasch K, Abhyankar B, Bhayat F, Blake A, et al. Vedolizumab exposure in pregnancy: Outcomes from clinical studies in inflammatory bowel disease. Alimentary Pharmacology & Therapeutics. 2017;**45**(7):941-950

[67] Moens A, van der Woude CJ, Julsgaard M, et al. Pregnancy outcomes in inflammatory bowel disease patients treated with vedolizumab, anti-TNF or conventional therapy: Results of the European CONCEIVE study. Alimentary Pharmacology & Therapeutics. 2020;**51**(1):129-138

[68] Moens A, van Hoeve K, Humblet E, Rahier JF, Bossuyt P, Dewit S, et al. Belgian IBD Research and Development group (BIRD). Outcome of Pregnancies in Female Patients With Inflammatory Bowel Diseases Treated With Vedolizumab. Journal of Crohn's and Colitis. 2019;**13**(1):12-18. DOI: 10.1093/ecco-jcc/jjy142. PMID: 30281093

[69] Flanagan E, Prentice R, Wright EK, Gibson PR, Ross AL, Begun J, et al. Ustekinumab levels in pregnant women with inflammatory bowel disease and infants exposed in utero. Alimentary Pharmacology & Therapeutics. 2022;**55**(6):700-704

[70] Nguyen GC, Seow CH, Maxwell C, Huang V, Leung Y, Jones J, et al. The Toronto consensus statements for the Management of Inflammatory Bowel Disease in pregnancy. Gastroenterology. 2016;**150**:734-757.e1

[71] Shi HY, Chan FK, Higashimori A, Chan A, Ching J, Wu JC, et al. Tu1949

Fecal calprotectin below 50ug/g predicts histologic remission: A prospective cohort study in quiescent ulcerative colitis. Gastroenterology. 1 Apr 2016;**150**(4):S987

[72] Harbord M, Eliakim R, Bettenworth D, Karmiris K, Katsanos K, Kopylov U, et al. European Crohn's and Colitis Organisation [ECCO], Third European Evidence-based Consensus on Diagnosis and Management of Ulcerative Colitis. Part 2: Current Management, Journal of Crohn's and Colitis. 2017;**11**(7):769-784. DOI: 10.1093/ecco-jcc/jjx009

[73] Ko MS, Rudrapatna VA, Avila P, Mahadevan U. Safety of flexible sigmoidoscopy in pregnant patients with known or suspected inflammatory bowel disease. Digestive Diseases and Sciences. 2020;**65**(10):2979-2985

[74] Brandt LJ, Estabrook SG, Reinus JF. Results of a survey to evaluate whether vaginal de- livery and episiotomy lead to perineal involvement in women with Crohn's disease. The American Journal of Gastroenterology. 1995;**90**:1918-1922

[75] Cornish JA, Tan E, Teare J, Teoh TG, Rai R, Darzi AW, et al. The effect of restorative proc-tocolectomy on sexual function, urinary function, fertility, pregnancy and delivery: A systematic review. Diseases of the Colon and Rectum. 2007;**50**(8):1128-1138

[76] Cheng K, Faye AS. Venous thromboembolism in inflammatory bowel disease. World Journal of Gastroenterology. 2020;**26**(12):1231-1241

[77] Seirafi M, de Vroey B, Amiot A, Seksik P, et al. Factors associated with pregnancy outcome in anti-TNF treated women with inflammatory bowel disease. Alimentary Pharmacology & Therapeutics. 2014;**40**(4):363-373

[78] Palomba S, Sereni G, Falbo A, Beltrami M, Lombardini S, Boni MC, et al. Inflammatory bowel diseases and human reproduction: A comprehensive evidence-based review. World Journal of Gastroenterology. 2014;**20**(23):7123-7136

[79] Mahadevan U, Robinson C, Bernasko N, et al. In- flammatory bowel disease in pregnancy clinical care pathway: A report from the American Gastroenterological Association IBD parenthood project working group. Inflammatory Bowel Diseases. 2019;**25**(4):627-641

[80] Johnson E, Carlsen E, Nazir M, Nygaard K. Morbidity and functional outcome after restorative proctocolectomy for ulcerative colitis. The European Journal of Surgery. 2001;**167**(1):40-45

[81] Roy A, Chambers CD, Martin C, Kane SV, Dubinsky M, Sandborn WJ, et al. Exposure to biologic therapy and childhood development among offspring of women with inflammatory bowel disease: Results from the Piano Registry. Gastroenterology. 2017;**152**:S85-S86

[82] Xu L, Lochhead P, Ko Y, Claggett B, Leong RW, Ananthakrishnan AN. Systematic review with meta-analysis: Breastfeeding and the risk of Crohn's disease and ulcerative colitis. Alimentary Pharmacology & Therapeutics. 2017;**46**(9):780-789

[83] National Library of Medicine. ToxNet. Toxicology Network. Available from: https://toxnet.nlm.nih.gov/pda/lactmed.htm [Accessed: December 7, 2021]

[84] Cleary BJ, Källén B. Early pregnancy azathi- oprine use and pregnancy outcomes. Birth Defects Research. Part A, Clinical and Molecular Teratology. 2009;**85**(7):647-654

[85] Matro R, Martin CF, Wolf D, Shah SA, Mahadevan U. Exposure concentrations

of In- fants breastfed by women receiving biologic therapies for inflammatory bowel diseases and effects of breastfeeding on infections and development. Gastroenterology. 2018;**155**(3):696-704

[86] Julsgaard M, Kjeldsen J, Bibby BM, Brock B, Baumgart DC. Vedolizumab concentrations in the breast Milk of nursing mothers with inflammatory bowel disease. Gastroenterology. 2018;**154**(3):752-4.e1

[87] Kane S, Lemieux N. The role of breastfeeding in postpartum disease activity in women with inflammatory bowel disease. The American Journal of Gastroenterology. 2005;**100**(1):102-105

[88] Moller FT, Andersen V, Wohlfahrt J, Jess T. Familial risk of inflammatory bowel disease: A population-based cohort study 1977-2011. The American Journal of Gastroenterology. 2015;**110**(4):564-571

[89] Mahadevan U, Robinson C, Bernasko N, Bo Johnson E, Carlsen E, Nazir M, et al. Morbidity and functional outcome after re- storative proctocolectomy for ulcerative coli- tis. The European Journal of Surgery. 2001;**167**(1):40-45

[90] Mahadevan U, Martin C, Chambers C, Kane SV, Dubinsky M, Sandborn W, et al. Achievement of developmental milestones among offspring of women with inflammatory bowel disease: The PIANO registry [abstract]. Gastroenterology. 2014;**146**(5):146

Section 5

Dietary Therapy

Chapter 8

Dietary Fermented Rice Bran Is an Effective Modulator of Ulcerative Colitis in Experimental Animal

Afroza Sultana, Abul Fazal Mohammad Nazmus Sadat and Md. Alauddin

Abstract

Ulcerative colitis (UC) is an inflammatory disorder with colon and rectum, characterized by recurring bloody diarrhea due to microbial dysfunction and some autoimmune response. Scientists have linked microbial disruption in the gut to several chronic conditions such as UC and other types of inflammatory bowel disease (IBD). Surprisingly, our gastrointestinal tract contains more than 100 trillion microbial cells. Some microbes in the gut microbiome are friendly bacteria that can help to treat UC by influencing metabolism, nutrition, immune function, and more in the gut. The conventional medical treatment of UC relies on the use of amino-salicylates, corticosteroids, immunosuppressive drugs, glucocorticoids, and antibiotics. Multiple new mechanisms in the treatment of UC are being developed and many are showing promising results in ulcerative colitis. Still need scientific evidence to support the role of gut microbiota in the etiology of UC. The dietary fermented rice bran (DFRB) may include the active potential for the treatment of ulcerative colitis. The DFRB may attenuate intestinal inflammation by regulating gut permeability for cellular infiltration and maintenance of luminal safety with favorable efficacy in UC. In this chapter, we discussed and summarized the insight mechanism of DFRB's modulatory activities for the management or treatment of ulcerative colitis.

Keywords: ulcerative colitis, fermented rice bran, gut microbiome, intestinal homeostasis, and tight junction barrier integrity

1. Introduction

Chronic inflammatory disease, ulcerative colitis (UC) is recognized by the luminal abnormalities by the flourishing of cytokines at the large intestine that can cause irritable mucosal lining cells and disruption of tight junction protein [1]. UC is one form of inflammatory bowel disease (IBD) and the severity was first coined in the 18th century [2]. Another form of this (IBD) disease is known as Crohn disease (CD). Worldwide, both diseases are commonly termed IBD and the frequency of this disease is observed commonly not only in the first world countries but also increasing this scenario in Asian countries due to their dietary habits. Surprisingly, the severity of this disease was found more common in Caucasians than other racial and colors people based on their lifestyle and food habits and as well as remarkably increased in Jewish [3]. The disease severity was found to be age dependent and the onset of the disease is 30–40 years old among the men and women equally [4]. The complexity of this disease makes a debilitating disorder by the discontinuous lacerations in the gut mucosal cell [5]. But the mechanism of inflammation in UC is typically confined in the mucosal cell lining that is the main cause of damage of the bowel wall and ultimately loss of mucosal tight barrier in the intestinal tract [6]. This mechanism has occurred recurrently in the mucosal cell lining leading to bloody diarrhea, which is the most common symptom of UC, although diagnosis is made from a combination of symptoms, endoscopy and histology [6]. The common symptom of UC is not only diarrhea with the blood but also some other symptoms sometimes less found with abdominal pain, body temperature, and weight loss [7]. The different types of UC can be recognized by the extent of the disease such as proctitis, this type of UC is limited to the end of the colon. Proctosigmoiditis is found in the rectum and sigmoid colon. The left-sided and extensive colitis is confined to and beyond splenic flexure [6, 8, 9]. The disease severity of UC is categorized as mild, moderate, severe, and fulminant with stool output category. If the stool output frequency is four per day with or without bloody is called mild, and more than four bloody stools per day is called moderate, more than six bloody stools per day is called severe and more than 10 bloody bowel movements with abdominal distention is called serious or fulminant colitis. UC disrupts not only the intestinal integrity but also predominantly affects the immunologic skin, joining part of the body, vision of eyes, and the most important organ liver [1, 6, 8, 9]. Similarly, different arthritis such as peripheral or axial and narrowing bile duct disease are also accompanying UC [1, 9]. The consequence of pathologic outcome for UC depends on dietary habits and environmental factors that can affect the host immunologic response, and ultimately change the microbiota symbiotic action in hereditarily vulnerable characters [10]. Dietary habits with lower fiber-based processed food and fewer intake of plant-based meals in lifestyle could be attributed to the augmented incidence of UC in the Asian population. A recent review article showed that the risk of UC is inversely associated with the herbal intake, they also found that the risk of UC is directly associated with total fat intake including Omega-6 fatty acids and meat [11].

In that connection food supplements are the important modulators of UC. The dietary habit with high fiber, multivitamins, free amino acids, bioactive compounds for antioxidants may be considered as the effective potential to encourage digestive health [12].

2. Etiology of ulcerative colitis

Even while its specific cause is still unknown, various contributing variables have been implicated such as an immunological response that is out of control, altered gut microbiota, genetic susceptibility, and environmental factors. The etiology of UC is primarily initiated by the invasion of inflammatory molecules to the intestinal tract changing the microbiota and ultimately loss of intestinal integrity causing bloody diarrhea [13]. The actual pathophysiologic pathway of UC remains elusive, but the number of studies postulated that overstimulation of immunologic function and insufficient control of mucosal barrier integrity leads to cell infiltration and inflammation in the intestinal tract [3]. The gastrointestinal tract is the main part of the body for digestion, absorption metabolism, and control of immunity for normal health. Disruption of this pathway may affect the deregulation of microbiota and mucosal immunological function is the main cause of propagation of UC [14, 15]. Deregulation of normal microbiota may change the pro-inflammatory molecules such as tumor necrosis factor α (TNF-α), interleukin 1β (IL-1β), and IL-6, which are responsible for colonic tissue damage and gut bleeding leading to ulceration of the colon. The intestinal tract contains a lot of microorganisms called microbiota, primarily bacteria; some other organisms including viruses, archaea, and fungi are responsible for inhibiting the gastrointestinal tract [16]. For example, the proteobacteria phylum, among other bacterial species, have been demonstrated as microbial initials in inflammatory bowel disease (IBD) for gut microbiota in IBD patients [17]. The non-eligible function of proteobacteria has been found for the development of IBD. The proteobacteria such as *E. coli*, was found to be disproportionately proliferated leading to the development of IBD [18]. This bacterial proliferation may influence the infiltration of severe and continuing provocative cells in the intestinal lumen. This provocative infiltration predominantly increases the mucosal immunoglobulin G production, subsequently chemoattractant complement activation leading to aggregation, and ultimately enhancement of macrophages and T cells. This cascade of immunological activity is connected with the discharge of inflammatory cytokines, kinins, leukotrienes, platelet-activating factor (PAF), and reactive oxygen metabolites in the gastrointestinal tract for initiation of IBD. The mechanism of these mediators that amplify the immune and inflammatory response not only the main cause but also have deviating effects on epithelial cell function which may increase the permeability, this is the cause of ischemia The mediators may influence on repair mechanisms in the colon, thus increasing the biosynthesis of collagen leading to the fibrosis process in the intestine, one of the causes of the intestinal bleeding. In addition, the acute phase striking forces such as IL-1, IL-6, and TNF-α will activate a chronic response in the intestinal lumen and ultimately. The resulting storm can cause fever in the body with an increased level of serum acute-phase proteins [19–22]. The detailed mechanism of intestinal increased permeability due to the cytokines storm is not completely stated, but an association with increased permeability due to the bacterial translocation into the lamina propria that could exacerbate the loss of tight junction protein and loss of barrier function [20].

3. Summary of possible mechanisms of UC treatment pathway

As the detailed mechanism of UC disease is unclear, so that there are no known single preventive or curative interventions or safe colectomy therapy was found in most of the IBD patients for lifelong [21]. Up to date most of the therapeutic treatments are able to inhibit the beginning of immunological and inflammatory effectors, loss of integrity protein, regulation of inflammatory cytokines, and loss of intestinal barrier mechanisms. These therapeutic strategies may lead to an improvement in the patient's symptoms and decrease inflammatory activity [1]. Several functional compounds and their metabolites may inhibit the UC progression. **Table 1** and **Figure 1** describe the possible mechanisms of UC treatment pathways that are commonly observed in the dextran sulfate sodium (DSS)-induced UC animal model.

Sl. no	Target of the pathways	Functional compounds	Reference
1	By restoration of tight junction protein and maintenance of barrier function.	Omega-3 fatty acid	[20]
2	The activation of transcription factors (PPARγ), possibly inhibiting Nfκ-b transcriptional activity and iκ-b phosphorylation and ERK1/2 pathway.	Omega-3 fatty acid, naringin, fiber and polyphenols, evodiamine, magnolol, eupatilin, terpinen-4-ol and allyl isothiocynate.	[21–29]
3	Inhibition of AMP-activated protein kinase (AMPK)	Fiber and polyphenols of red raspberry Eupatilin (flavonoid) found in the leaves of Artemisia argyi	[24, 26]
4	Restoration of crypts losses	Magnolol from Magnolia officinalis Terpinen-4-ol from Zanthoxylum bungeanum.	[27, 28]
5	Suppression of oxidative stress enzyme such as NOs and COX-2.	Porcine β-defensine-2.	[30]
6	Inhibition of inflammatory cytokines IL-1,IL-1β, IL-6,TNF-α.	short-chain fatty acid such as propionate and antimicrobial peptide like Porcine βdefensine-2	[30–32]
7	Reduced the infiltration of neutrophil.	short-chain fatty acid such as propionate and antimicrobial peptide like Porcine βdefensine-2	[30–32]
8	Inhibition of paracellular migration.	short-chain fatty acid	[32]
9	Reduce epithelial hyper permeability by regulating occluding, ZO-1 ZO-2, claudin1 and E-cadherin junctional adhesion molecule-A (JAM-A), claudin-3, claudin-4, claudin-7, mucin.	short peptide such as Chromofungin, naringin, fiber and polyphenols.	[10, 23, 24, 30, 33–40]
10	Inhibited oxidative stress	Phloretin (a flavonoid available in apples and strawberries)	[34]
11	Ameliorate colitis by regulation of IL-8 and STAT3	Chromofungin	[35]
12	Reduce colon tissue damage	Neuropeptides.	[38]
13	Down regulation of IL-8 and STAT3	Catestin	[39, 40]
14	Inhibited the loss of goblet cells	Phloretin (a flavonoid available in apples and strawberries) Phellinus igniarius (medicinal mushroom) Terpinen-4-ol from zanthoxylum bungeanum Allyl isothiocynate from wasabia japonica	[27, 29, 34, 41]
15	Stabilized intercellular junctions by regulating IL-10	Oleanolic acid	[29, 32, 35]
16	Inhibition of the NLRP3 inflammasome	Phloretin (a flavonoid available in apples and strawberries) Formononetin is a natural isoflavone Evodiamine (an alkaloid obtained from Evodia rutaecarpa) Terpinen-4-ol from Zanthoxylum bungeanum	[25, 27, 34, 36]

Sl. no	Target of the pathways	Functional compounds	Reference
17	Inhibit histological damage	Salvianolic acid a (phenolic compound) found in salvia miltiorrhiza bunge (danshen)	[37]
18	Inhibit leukocyte infiltration	Salvianolic acid a (phenolic compound) found in salvia miltiorrhiza bunge (danshen) Magnolol from magnolia officinalis	[28, 37]
19	Protected against weight loss and colon shortening	Antrum mucosa peptide (amp-18)	[42]
20	Regulation of microbiota in UC patients.	Escherichia coli strain Nissle 1917.	[43]
21	Controlling inflammation by regulating innate and adaptive immune responses	Vitamin d and its receptor	[44]
22	Direct scavenging of reactive oxygen species	Curcumin, a polyphenolic antioxidant	[45]
23	Ameliorate colonic inflammatory responses by modulates mucosal permeability.	Aloe anthraquinones and chromone	[20, 46]
24	Regulation of phase-II-detoxifying enzymes.	Moringa isothiocyanates	[41]
25	Inhibition of bacterial translocation	Isoflavonoids from soybeans and barley	[47]
26	Inhibit edema in the mouse colon	Salvianolic acid a (phenolic compound) found in salvia miltiorrhiza bunge	[37, 48]

Table 1.
Prospective pathways and modulators for minimizing UC (revised from the experiment on dextran sulfate sodium (DSS) induced UC animal).

4. Dietary fermented rice bran (DFRB) as an alternative modulator for ulcerative colitis treatment

The by-product of the rice grain is called rice bran (RB) a valuable and low costing source of biologically active components that is currently available in most regions of the world. It has been possible to improve the quality or make RB edible for humans by using RB procedures such as bacterial fermentation. In contrast to typical raw bran, treated RB or nutritionally enriched dietary fermented rice bran (DFRB) include more basic nutrients such as proximate composition and bioactive compounds [49]. Rice bran is one of the most plentiful agricultural products in Asian countries and is a superb source of nutritional fiber, protein, and fat [50]. RB has been recently claimed for its nutraceutical properties; specific components of the lipid fraction of RB such as tocotrienols, a group of compounds with vitamin E [51]. The difficulty of its use is because of its excessive fiber content material, low protein, and antinutritional elements along with phytic acid [52]. Most of the dietary fiber content in RB belongs to the class of insoluble dietary fiber which may be beneficial for increasing fecal bulk and laxation [53].

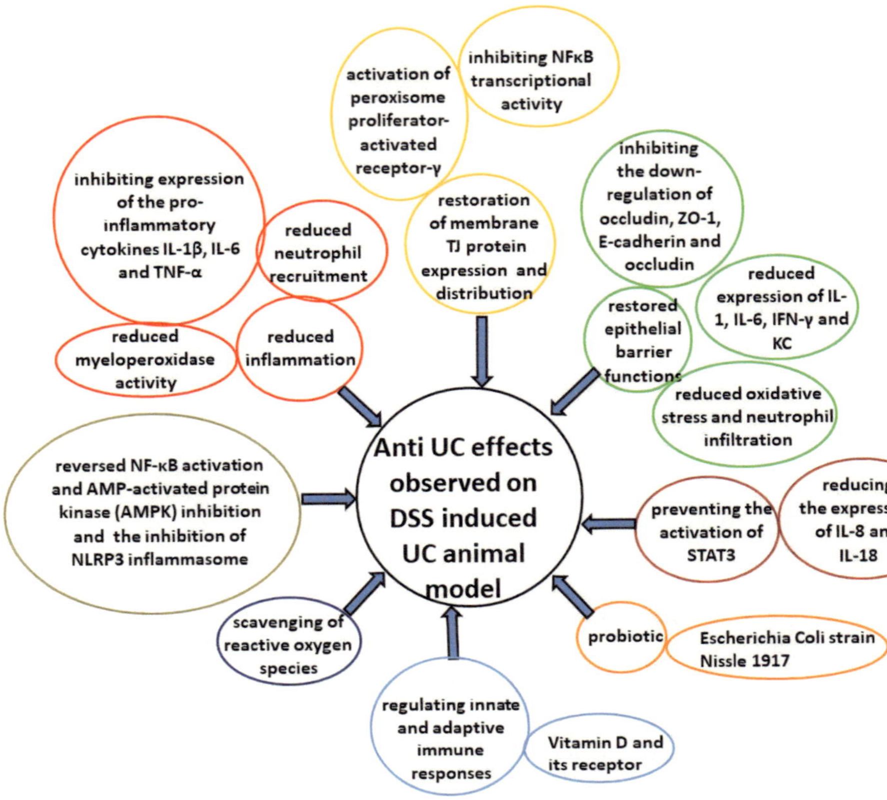

Figure 1.
Anti ulcerative effects observed in experimental animal.

4.1 Nutritionally enriched dietary fermented rice bran

Recent studies have suggested that fermentation can improve their biological activities. Fermenting is the process of naturally gathering wild cultures and yeasts from the air and combining them with an organic substance. During the fermentation process, sugars and starches contained in the feed ingredients are broken down into lactic acid bacteria (LAB). The lactic acid formed by the action of LAB from substrate sugars through pyruvate (a glycolysis end product) plays an important role in food fermentation. Fermentation technology produces not only lactic acid, but also other end products such as ethanol, acetic acid, and formic acid depending on bacterial species and conditions [54]. The lactic acid bacteria produced during fermentation promote the growth of beneficial microbes called probiotics. These improve the digestive system health and boost the immune system. Feed fermentation is a complex process that depends on the nutritional requirements and digestive physiology of animals, the nutritive value of feedstuffs, fermentation characteristics of the microorganisms added to the starter culture, and actual situations on individual farms [55]. Systematic use of bacteria may improve desired food ingredients in the diet.

Previous studies reported that *Bacillus amyloliquefaciens* may successfully produce various enzymes such as αamylase, α-acetolactate, decarboxylase, β-endoglucanase, hemicellulase, phytase, maltogenic amylase, and xylanase, which possess the potential to degrade fiber [56]. Some lactic acid bacterial strains can produce Exopolysaccharides (EPS), which exert health-promoting effects as a function of prebiotics. The EPS may be responsible for the immunomodulator action [53]. Due to the significant increment of protein content in the fermented rice bran, the quality of this produced compound is the target of interest. Dietary fermented rice bran (DFRB) has been interested in particular for the treatment of unfavorable duodenal inflammation. DFRB supplementation would be able to alter intestinal inflammation caused by DSS-induced colitis. The evidence of DFRB was found to raise the amounts of striking modulators such as short-chain fatty acids and other microbial metabolites in the gastrointestinal tract. Tryptamine is one of them which comes from tryptophan metabolism in the intestine by beneficial microorganisms. The striking modulator metabolites may regulate the intestinal loss of tight junction barrier and ultimately intestinal microbiota homeostasis. The preventive action of DFRB may be partially due to the availability of bioactive compounds during fermentation of rice bran, such as polysaccharides, carbohydrate conjugated proteins, γ-oryzanol, plant sterols, and antioxidant vitamin E. DFRB is very important for the regulation of IBD patients because of fermentation technique make its bioactive compounds more accessible and easier to metabolize. Several studies have pointed out that fermentation technologies enhance the amount of the total phenolic content, short-chain fatty acids, amino acids, and other metabolites that can ameliorate intestinal inflammation. Consequently, it is prospective that DFRB can be used not only as a protective measure but also as a beneficial mediator against an ongoing intestinal inflammation like UC [49, 57–60].

4.2 DFRB as ulcerative colitis modulator

One of the enriched ingredients of DFRB is tryptamine, 5-hydroxytryptamine comes out as bacterial metabolites. These metabolites are considered an effective modulators for the candidate against UC [7, 14]. Tryptophan, one of the boosted constituents in DFRB, is recognized as an effective modulator for UC [7, 14]. Tryptamine and 5-hydroxytryptamine derived from tryptophan, can act as a ligand for the receptor of the aryl hydrocarbon, which modulates immunologic cytokines IL-22 gene production, controls autoimmune, and facilitates fast recovery from colitis in the large intestine. Some insoluble DFRB may also stimulate the microbial proliferation and production of short-chain fatty acids (SCFAs), particularly, acetic acid (AA), propionic acid (PA), butyric acid (BA), and lactic acid (LA), which are strappingly linked with the colonic health in DSS induced UC [15, 49].

A single modulator for the treatment of IBD seems difficult to pinpoint due to the intricate interplay of various variables. For individuals with IBD, the use of biologically effective significant functional compounds such as anti-tumor necrosis factor (TNF) drugs have lowered early surgery. Nevertheless, there are still many difficulties with current treatment intervention and new therapies are highly required. In various experimental murine colitis models, many single substances or combinations made from natural commodities based on traditional usage knowledge have shown promising anti-inflammatory qualities with minimal negative effects and have the potential to be next-generation therapeutics. Even now, clinical studies are being conducted on several plants' small components, including berberine, curcumin, epigallocatechin-3-gallate (EGCG), and triptolide. There is a new IBD treatment in the works, a recovered anti-mycobacterium drug (Oral capsule RHB-104, here, RHB-104 = Red hill biopharma, an investigational drug), now in phase III clinical trials. The current therapy challenges associated with numerous side effects might be greatly improved by using a suitable and non-invasive IBD medication that targets specific receptors in the colon. Ethnopharmacology-guided drug discovery, with a particular emphasis on tiny molecules and peptides of medicinal plants, has the potential to generate safe and new therapies for IBD. Clinical and histological damage to the colon is both reduced by a cardiotrophin (CT)-1 injection before DSS induction. This effect seems to be done by inhibiting inflammation and apoptosis directly and activating the Stat-3 and nuclear factor kappa B (NF-kB) signaling pathways. Stat-3 and NF-kB CT-1 might potentially be expected to be a feasible, innovative method to prevent UC relapse. A fermented diet was included in the regular diet as a supplement. When given a Fermented diet (FD) with DSS for 7 days, mice did not lose weight or suffer from atrophy of the intestinal length. IL-6 and TNF-_ levels in the mice did not rise after FD treatment, indicating that inflammation was kept under control. People who ate an FPE-enriched diet for 3 months had an increased clostridiales order in their feces, which generates short-chain fatty acids to reduce inflammation. FPE supplementation has been shown to increase the proliferation of Clostridiales in the gut, as well as to reduce inflammation in colitis [61–63].

Another research found that the relative abundance of bacteroidetes species was adversely associated with UC activity and might serve as important microbiological biomarkers to monitor UC disease activity and exacerbation. A reliable and non-invasive method for monitoring UC and establishing personalized therapy might be made possible by identifying components of the microbiome that are associated with disease activity. In mice with inflamed intestines, FRB supplementation helped to heal the damage caused by DSS. DAI scores and the generation of intestinal pro-inflammatory cytokines were reduced by FRB administration. The anti-inflammatory cytokine Il-10, the tight junction component Clad4, and antimicrobial proteins were all considerably increased by FRB supplementation in the gut. This capacity to inhibit both canonical and non-canonical pathways of Tgf-b profibrogenic activity was also able to reduce the development of fibrosis in mice intestines after inflammation. Using FRB supplements to reduce inflammation is not the only way to repair the intestines in people with chronic colitis, according to the findings of this study. It has been postulated that FRB acts as a prebiotic in the gut, but even if intestinal dysbiosis has developed as a result of inflammation, it may still treat colitis. As a result, the role of FRB supplementation on gut microbiota populations and composition has to be studied further [63–65].

In **Figure 2,** three different conditions of intestinal luminal microbial flora. The movement of luminal microbiota and smoothie mucosal protection has been seen in stage 1, generally is regulated by pro-inflammatory cytokines such as IL-10,IL-1β, IL-4,IL-6,TNF-α, and membrane tight junction protein occludin, ZO-1 and E-cadherin etc. indicate normal expression of cell. In stage 2, the changed luminal microbial diversity (dysbiosis), impaired epithelial, and mucus layer barrier via disruption of tight junctions expressed the intestinal inflammation mediated by Dextran sodium sulfate (DSS). Usually, DSS induced inflammation prompts to disruption of the mucosal layer, with an increased loss of crypts, inflammatory cell infiltration, increased MPO activity, and pro-inflammatory cytokine transcript (Tnf- α, Il-1 β, Il-6, and Il-17) associated with excessive intestinal epithelial permeability via the tight junction of epithelial and by increasing luminal antigen uptaking. That's how Toll-like receptors recognize non-pathogenic bacteria (commensal microbiota) and activate antigen-presenting cell (e.g. TLRs) APC activated T-cells become Th-2 effector cells (which produce

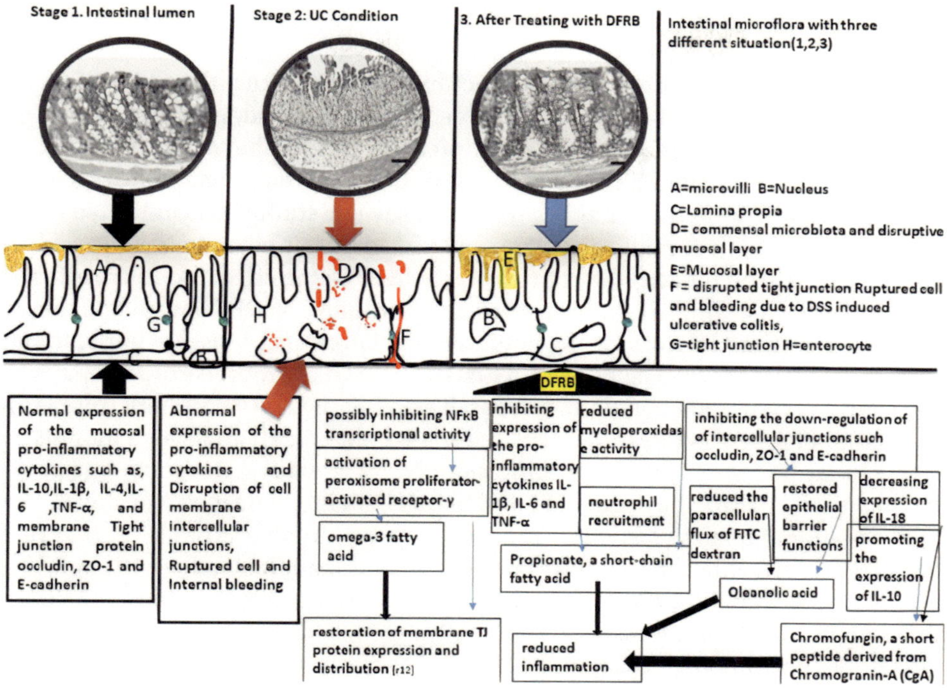

Figure 2.
A simple fictional image of enterocytes associated with normal behavior, inflammatory condition and after treatment with DFRB (review from [62, 67]).

pro-inflammatory cytokines like TNF-, IL-5, IL-6, and IL-13). TNF and IL-1 activate the NF-B pathway, promoting pro-inflammatory and cell survival genes.

The mucin generation and epithelium integrity appeared in the 3rd stage of this fictional image of intestinal lumen after treating with DFRB and it has been proved by Islam (2017) that, this incidence is facilitated by increased SCFA levels in the colon via inducing colonic regulatory T cells and reducing UC. Also, apoptosis can be induced in mutated epithelial cells through innate immune cell-driven inflammation. To maintain colonic homeostasis and intestinal barrier integrity, these activities are essential. Thus, the integrity of the intestinal barrier helps not only to maintain a healthy relationship between the intestinal microbes and the host but in addition to being a physical barrier, it also serves as a barrier to the entry of invading microorganisms pathogenic microorganisms or their toxins can be detected by an organism's immune system. Tight junctions (TJs) are made up of occludin and a variety of other proteins (OCLN) and claudin (CLDN), which are primarily responsible for determining the integrity of the intestinal barrier. TJs can be found here. At the ends of the epithelial cell's lateral membrane, the loss of TJ barrier integrity is linked to the onset and progression of UC.

The study has shown that transcription factor named by aryl hydrocarbon receptor (Ahr) regulates the expression of IL-22 genes, controls autoimmunity processes, and promotes rapid recovery from colitis by binding to tryptophan-metabolites in the microbiota. DFRB might boost up the microbial power generation of short-chain fatty acids (SCFAs), such as AA, PA, BA, LA, which are intimately connected to colonic health of us, might even be a result of DFRB [61, 66].

5. Future perspective

A number of fermentation studies on rice bran indicated that the process is capable of producing short-chain fatty acids such as acetic acid, propionic acid, butyric acid, lactic acid, enzymes such as protease amylase, phenolic compound, and antioxidant compound like vitamin E as well as secondary metabolites such as griseofulvin, etc. for treatment of UC [67–74]. Previous studies also indicated that it is possible to change the lipid and phospholipid composition and phenolic acid content and antioxidant activities of rice bran would be the effect modulators for the treatment of UC [75, 76]. In the future, the possibility of DFRB would be the natural source of modulators for the potential regulators of the disease burden. The single-component of DFRB such as short-chain fatty (like Propionate), omega-3 fatty acid (like eicosapentaenoic and docosahexaenoic acid), fibers (both soluble and insoluble), polyphenols (oleanolic acid and salvianolic acids), and even vitamins (C, D, E) may be responsible for specific modulators in the maintenance of gastro-intestinal tract health. The detailed experimental data is still needed worldwide. These vibrant modulators could be produced by using suitable variants of bacteria and fungi for fermentation as well as by using recombinant technology to modify the bacteria and fungi for a specific purpose. However, variations in the conformation of duodenal microorganisms are generally responsible for the establishment of gut health in patients with UC. Furthermore, DFRB influences not only the attendance of gastric microbiota but also modulates their metabolites. The interchange of microbes and metabolites by the DFRB would be a good modulator to alter the intestinal defense mechanism against mucosal inflammation for the treatment of UC [23]. The DFRB also modulates impaired DNA integrity that occurs during oxidation after the intestinal inflammation [24]. Hence, the DFRB would be a good candidate for therapeutic treatment of UC rather than a preventive measure, but this scenario still requires many animal experiments. This is a significant peculiarity of DFRB to make a potential modulator, especially in the case of IBD. Whereas the treatments of IBD are generally aimed to prevent a flare-up of enduring inflammation and to hinder its development into an irreversible state such as stricture and altered colonic motility and permeability [66].

6. Conclusions

The availability of bioactive components in DFRB, such as dietary fiber, vitamins, free amino acids, and antioxidants, ensures the potential of DFRB to improve the health of the gastrointestinal tract (gastrointestinal health). By utilizing fermentation technology, it is possible to incorporate many more nutrients into rice bran, particularly potential UC modulators, than are currently available. The nutritional content of rice bran is typically determined by the fermented organism, the length of time the bran has been fermented, and the source or types of rice bran used. A high level of concentration is required to isolate the specific bacteria, fungi, or yeast that is capable of producing the desired fatty acids, fibers, vitamins, amino acids, anti-inflammatory, antioxidants, and other compounds in fermented rice bran. Using recombinant technology, it may be possible to produce the desired microorganisms for use in the fermentation process, which would then be used to introduce desired nutrition into the DFRB. This will also be beneficial in the treatment of other metabolic conditions in addition to UC colitis.

Acknowledgements

I am particularly grateful to Jashore University of Science and Technology for the logistic support of this cha–pter.

Authors contribution

Md. Alauddin conceived the study design and manuscript preparation. AFM Nazmus Sadat carried out suggestions and data analysis. All the authors contributed to analysis and Afroza sultana contributed to manuscript writing. Md. Alauddin approved the final version of the manuscript.

Conflict of interest

The authors declare no conflict of interest.

Appendices and nomenclature

UC	Ulcerative colitis
IBD	Inflammatory bowel disease
DFRB	Dietary fermented rice bran
CD	Crohn disease
TNF-α	Tumor necrosis factor α
L-1β	Interleukin 1beta
IL-6	Interleukin 6
PAF	Platelet-activating factor
DSS	Dextran sulfate sodium
NF-kB	Nuclear factor kappa B
AMPK	AMP-activated protein kinase
FITC dextran	Fluorescein isothiocyanates–dextran
Zo	tight junction protein
JAM-A	E-cadherin junctional adhesion molecule-A
STAT3	Signal transducer and activator of transcription 3, transcription factor
LAB	Lactic acid bacteria
EPS	Exopolysaccharides
Ahr	Aryl hydrocarbon receptor
Profibrogenic cytokine e.g. TGF-β1.	
SMDs	Small-molecule medicines (such as tofacitinib and 5-ASA derivatives mesalamine)
Tj	Tight junction
AA	Acetic acid
PA	Propanoic acid
BA	Butyl acid

Author details

Afroza Sultana[1], Abul Fazal Mohammad Nazmus Sadat[2] and Md. Alauddin[1*]

1 Department of Nutrition and Food Technology, Jashore University of Science and Technology, Jashore, Bangladesh

2 Institute of Environmental Science, Rajshahi University, Rajshahi, Bangladesh

*Address all correspondence to: mdalauddin1181@gmail.com

References

[1] Feuerstein JD, Cheifetz AS. Ulcerative colitis. Mayo Clinic Proceedings. 2014; **89**(11):1553-1563

[2] Kirsner JB. Historical origins of current IBD concepts. World Journal of Gastroenterology. 2001;7(2):175

[3] Ardizzone S, Cassinotti A, Duca P, Mazzali C, Penati C, Manes G, et al. Mucosal healing predicts late outcomes after the first course of corticosteroids for newly diagnosed ulcerative colitis. Clinical Gastroenterology and Hepatology. 2011;**9**(483-489):e3. DOI: 10.1016/j.cgh.2010.12.028

[4] Cosnes J, Gower-Rousseau C, Seksik P, Cortot A. Epidemiology and natural history of inflammatory bowel diseases. Gastroenterology. 2011;**140**:1785-1794

[5] Da Silva C, Lyra AC, Rocha R, Santana GO. Epidemiology, demographic characteristics, and prognostic predictors of ulcerative colitis. World Journal of Gastroenterology. 2014;**28**:9458-9467

[6] Kobayashi T, Siegmund B, Le Berre C, et al. Ulcerative colitis. Nature Reviews. Disease Primers. 2020;**6**:74. DOI: 10.1038/s41572-020-0205-x

[7] Huang B, Kwan LY, Shih DQ. Extraintestinal manifestations of ulcerative colitis. In: Ulcerative Colitis-Epidemiology, Pathogenesis and Complications. London: IntechOpen; 2011. DOI: 10.5772/26042

[8] Ford AC, Moayyedi P, Hanauer SB. Ulcerative colitis. BMJ. 2013;**346**:432. DOI: 10.1136/bmj.f432

[9] Kornbluth A, Sachar DB. Ulcerative colitis practice guidelines in adults. American Journal of Gastroenterology. 1997;**92**(2):204-211

[10] Ungaro R, Mehandru S, Alle PB, Peyrin-Biroulet L, Colombel JF. Ulcerative colitis. Lancet. 2017;**389**: 1756-1770

[11] Hou JK, Abraham B, El-Serag H. Dietary intake and risk of developing inflammatory bowel disease: A systematic review of the literature. The American Journal of Gastroenterology. 2011;**106**:563-573. DOI: 10.1038/ajg.2011.44

[12] Choi JY, Paik DJ, Kwon DY, Park Y. Dietary supplementation with rice bran fermented with Lentinus edodes increases interferon-γ activity without causing adverse effects: A randomized, double-blind, placebo-controlled, parallel-group study. The Journal of Nutrition. 2014;**13**:35

[13] Hibi T, Ogata H. Novel pathophysiological concepts of inflammatory bowel disease. Journal of Gastroenterology. 2006;**41**:10-16

[14] Rowland I, Gibson G, Heinken A, Scott K, Swann J, Thiele I, et al. Gut microbiota functions: Metabolism of nutrients and other food components. European Journal of Nutrition. 2018;**57**:1-24. DOI: 10.1007/s00394-017-1445-8

[15] Kataoka K, Ogasa S, Kuwahara T, Bando Y, Hagiwara M, Arimochi H, et al. Inhibitory effects of fermented brown rice on induction of acute colitis by dextran sulfate sodium in rats. Digestive Diseases and Sciences. 2008;**53**:1601-1608

[16] Yu LC. Microbiota dysbiosis and barrier dysfunction in inflammatory bowel disease and colorectal cancers: Exploring a common ground hypothesis. Journal of Biomedical Science. 2018;**25**:79. DOI: 10.1186/s12929-018-0483-8

[17] Mukhopadhya I, Hansen R, El-Omar EM, Hold GL. IBD-what role do proteobacteria play? Nature Reviews. Gastroenterology & Hepatology. 2012;**9**:219-230. DOI: 10.1038/nrgastro.2012.14

[18] Palmela C, Chevarin C, Xu Z, Torres J, Sevrin G, Hirten R, et al. Adherent-invasive Escherichia coli in inflammatory bowel disease. Gut. 2018;**67**(3):574-587

[19] Büning C, Geissler N, Prager M, Sturm A, Baumgart DC, Büttner J, et al. Increased small intestinal permeability in ulcerative colitis: Rather genetic than environmental and a risk factor for extensive disease? Inflammatory Bowel Diseases. 2012;**18**:1932-1939. DOI: 10.1002/ibd.22909

[20] Sung MK, Park MY. Nutritional modulators of ulcerative colitis: Clinical efficacies and mechanistic view. World Journal of Gastroenterology. 2013;**19**(7):994

[21] Kayal M, Shah S. Ulcerative colitis: Current and emerging treatment strategies. Journal of Clinical Medicine. 2020;**9**(1):94

[22] Toedter G, Li K, Sague S, Ma K, Marano C, Macoritto M, et al. Genes associated with intestinal permeability in ulcerative colitis: Changes in expression following infliximab therapy. Inflammatory Bowel Diseases. 2012;**18**:1399-1410. DOI: 10.1002/ibd.22853

[23] Cao H, Liu J, Shen P, Cai J, Han Y, Zhu K, et al. Protective effect of naringin on DSS-induced ulcerative colitis in mice. Journal of Agricultural and Food Chemistry. 2018;**66**(50):13133-13140

[24] Bibi S, Kang Y, Du M, Zhu MJ. Dietary red raspberries attenuate dextran sulfate sodium-induced acute colitis. Journal of Nutritional Biochemistry. 2018;**51**:40-46. DOI: 10.1016/j.jnutbio.2017.08.017

[25] Shen P, Zhang Z, Zhu K, Cao H, Liu J, Lu X, et al. Evodiamine prevents dextran sulfate sodium-induced murine experimental colitis via the regulation of NF-κB and NLRP3 inflammasome. Biomedicine & Pharmacotherapy. 2019;**110**:786-795. DOI: 10.1016/j.biopha.2018.12.033

[26] Zhou K, Cheng R, Liu B, Wang L, Xie H, Zhang C. Eupatilin ameliorates dextran sulphate sodium induced colitis in mice partly through promoting AMPK activation. Phytomedicine. 2018;**46**:46-56. DOI: 10.1016/j.phymed.2018.04.033

[27] Zhang Z, Shen P, Lu X, Li Y, Liu J, Liu B, et al. In vivo and in vitro study on the efficacy of terpinen-4-ol in dextran sulfate sodium-induced mice experimental colitis. Frontiers in Immunology. 2017;**12**(8):558

[28] Shen P, Zhang Z, He Y, Gu C, Zhu K, Li S, et al. Magnolol treatment attenuates dextran sulphate sodium-induced murine experimental colitis by regulating inflammation and mucosal damage. Life Sciences. 2018;**196**:69-76. DOI: 10.1016/j.lfs.2018.01.016

[29] Kim MW, Choi S, Kim SY, Yoon YS, Kang JH, Oh SH. Allyl isothiocyanate ameliorates dextran sodium sulfate-induced colitis in mouse by enhancing tight junction and mucin expression. International Journal of Molecular Sciences. 2018;**19**(7):2025

[30] Han F, Zhang H, Xia X, Xiong H, Song D, Zong X, et al. Porcine β-defensin 2 attenuates inflammation and mucosal lesions in dextran sodium sulfate-induced colitis. Journal of Immunology.

2015;**194**:1882-1893. DOI: 10.4049/jimmunol.1402300

[31] Tong LC, Wang Y, Wang ZB, Liu WY, Sun S, Li L, et al. Propionate ameliorates dextran sodium sulfate-induced colitis by improving intestinal barrier function and reducing inflammation and oxidative stress. Frontiers in Pharmacology. 2016;7:253

[32] Kang GD, Lim S, Kim DH. Oleanolic acid ameliorates dextran sodium sulfate-induced colitis in mice by restoring the balance of Th17/Treg cells and inhibiting NF-κB signaling pathway. International Immunopharmacology. 2015;**29**:393-400. DOI: 10.1016/j.intimp.2015.10.024

[33] Azuma T, Shigeshiro M, Kodama M, Tanabe S, Suzuki T. Supplemental naringenin prevents intestinal barrier defects and inflammation in colitic mice. Journal of Nutrition. 2013;**143**:827-834. DOI: 10.3945/jn.113.174508

[34] Zhang Z, Li S, Cao H, Shen P, Liu J, Fu Y, et al. The protective role of phloretin against dextran sulfate sodium-induced ulcerative colitis in mice. Food & Function. 2019;**10**:422-431. DOI: 10.1039/c8fo01699b

[35] Eissa N, Hussein H, Tshikudi DM, Hendy GN, Bernstein CN, Ghia JE. Interdependence between chromogranin-a, alternatively activated macrophages, tight junction proteins and the epithelial functions. A human and in-vivo/in-vitro descriptive study. International Journal of Molecular Sciences. 2020;**21**(21):7976

[36] Wu D, Wu K, Zhu Q, Xiao W, Shan Q, Yan Z, et al. Formononetin administration ameliorates dextran sulfate sodium-induced acute colitis by inhibiting NLRP3 inflammasome signaling pathway. Mediators of Inflammation. 2018;**2018**:3048532. DOI: 10.1155/2018/3048532

[37] Wang K, Yang Q, Ma Q, Wang B, Wan Z, Chen M, et al. Protective effects of salvianolic acid a against dextran sodium sulfate-induced acute colitis in rats. Nutrients. 2018;**10**:E791. DOI: 10.3390/nu10060791

[38] Hwang DY, Kim S, Hong HS. Substance-P ameliorates dextran sodium sulfate-induced intestinal damage by preserving tissue barrier function. Tissue Engineering and Regenerative Medicine. 2018;**15**(1):63-73

[39] Ogata M, Ogita T, Tari H, Arakawa T, Suzuki T. Supplemental psyllium fibre regulates the intestinal barrier and inflammation in normal and colitic mice. British Journal of Nutrition. 2017;**118**(9):661-672

[40] Eissa N, Hussein H, Mesgna R, Bonin S, Hendy GN, Metz-Boutigue MH, et al. Catestatin regulates epithelial cell dynamics to improve intestinal inflammation. Vaccine. 2018;**6**(4):67

[41] Kim Y, Wu AG, Jaja-Chimedza A, Graf BL, Waterman C, Verzi MP, et al. Isothiocyanate-enriched moringa seed extract alleviates ulcerative colitis symptoms in mice. PLoS One. 2017;**12**:e0184709. DOI: 10.1371/journal.pone.0184709

[42] Chen P, Bakke D, Kolodziej L, Lodolce J, Weber CR, Boone DL, et al. Antrum mucosal protein. Peptide targets tight junctions to protect and heal barrier structure and function in models of inflammatory bowel disease. Inflammatory Bowel Diseases. 2015;**21**:2393-2402. DOI: 10.1097/MIB.0000000000000499

[43] Trebichavsky I, Splichal I, Rada V, Splichalova A. Modulation of natural

immunity in the gut by Escherichia coli strain Nissle 1917. Nutrition Reviews. 2010;**68**(8):459-464

[44] Tabatabaeizadeh SA, Tafazoli N, Ferns GA, Avan A, Ghayour-Mobarhan M. Vitamin D, the gut microbiome and inflammatory bowel disease. Journal of Research in Medical Sciences. 2018;**23**:75. DOI: 10.4103/jrms.JRMS_606_17

[45] Holt PR, Katz S, Kirshoff R. Curcumin therapy in inflammatory bowel disease: A pilot study. Digestive Diseases and Sciences. 2005;**50**:2191-2193. DOI: 10.1007/s10620-005-3032-8

[46] Park MY, Kwon HJ, Sung MK. Dietary aloin, aloesin, or aloe-gel exerts anti-inflammatory activity in a rat colitis model. Life Sciences. 2011;**88**:486-492. DOI: 10.1016/j.lfs.2011.01.010

[47] Woo JK, Choi S, Kang JH, Kim DE, Hurh BS, Jeon JE, et al. Fermented barley and soybean (BS) mixture enhances intestinal barrier function in dextran sulfate sodium (DSS)-induced colitis mouse model. BMC Complementary and Alternative Medicine. 2016;**16**:498. DOI: 10.1186/s12906-016-1479-0

[48] Danese S, Fiocchi C. Ulcerative colitis. The New England Journal of Medicine. 2011;**365**(18):1713-1725

[49] Alauddin M, Shirakawa H, Koseki T, Kijima N, Ardiansyah; Budijanto, S, Islam, J, Goto, T, Komai, M. Fermented rice bran supplementation mitigates metabolic syndrome in stroke-prone spontaneously hypertensive rats. BMC Complementary and Alternative Medicine. 2016;**16**:1-11

[50] Prakash J. Rice bran proteins: Properties and food uses. Critical Reviews in Food Science and Nutrition. 1996;**36**(6):537-552. DOI: 10.1080/10408399609527738

[51] Sen CK, Khanna S, Roy S. Tocotrienols in health and disease: The other half of the natural vitamin E family. Molecular Aspects of Medicine. 2007;**28**:692-728

[52] Supriyati H, T. Susanti T. and Susan IW. Nutritional value of rice bran fermented by bacillus amyloliquefaciens and humic substances and its utilization as a feed ingredient for broiler chickens. Asian-Australasian Journal of Animal Sciences. 2015;**28**(2):231-238. DOI: 10.5713/ajas.14

[53] Murphy DCL, M R, and Fahey GC, Jr. Dietary fibers affect viscosity of solutions and simulated human gastric and small intestinal digesta. The Journal of Nutrition. 2006;**136**(4):913-919. DOI: 10.1093/jn/136.4.913

[54] Mozzi F. Lactic acid bacteria. Reference module in food science. In: Encyclopedia of Food and Health. Science Direct. 2016. pp. 501-508. DOI: 10.1016/B978-0-12-384947-2.00414-1

[55] Daia Z, Cuia L, Lib J, Wang B, Guo L, Wu Z, et al. Chapter 24- fermentation techniques in feed production. In: Animal Agriculture, Sustainability, Challenges and Innovations. London: Academic Press, Elsevier; 2020. pp. 407-429

[56] Diaz D. Safety and efficacy of Ecobiol® (bacillus amyloliquefaciens) as feed additive for chickens for fattening. European Food Safety Authority Journal. 2008;**773**:2-13

[57] Hefnawy HTM, El-shourbagy GA. Chemical analysis and antioxidant activity of polysaccharide extracted from rice bran. World Journal of Dairy & Food Sciences. 2014;**9**:95-104

[58] Park HY, Yu AR, Choi IW, Hong H, Lee KW, Choi HD. Immunostimulatory effects and characterization of a

glycoprotein fraction from rice bran. International Immunopharmacology. 2013;**17**:191-197

[59] Justo ML, Candiracci M, Dantas AP, de Sotomayor MA, Parrado J, Vila E, et al. Rice bran enzymatic extract restores endothelial function and vascular contractility in obese rats by reducing vascular inflammation and oxidative stress. Journal of Nutritional Biochemistry. 2013;**24**:1453-1461

[60] Rashid NYA, Razak DLA, Jamaluddin A, Sharifuddin SA, Long K. Bioactive compounds and antioxidant activity of rice bran fermented with lactic acid bacteria. Malaysian Journal of Microbiology. 2015;**11**:156-162

[61] Yeshi K, Ruscher R, Hunter L, Daly NL, Loukas A, Wangchuk P. Revisiting inflammatory bowel disease: Pathology, treatments, challenges and emerging therapeutics including drug leads from natural products. Journal of Clinical Medicine. 2020;**9**(5):1273

[62] Sánchez-Garrido AI, Prieto-Vicente V, Blanco-Gozalo V, Arévalo M, Quiros Y, López-Montañés D, et al. Preventive effect of cardiotrophin-1 administration before DSS-induced ulcerative colitis in mice. Journal of Clinical Medicine. 2019;**8**(12):2086

[63] Sugimoto M, Watanabe T, Takaoka M, Suzuki K, Murakami T, Murakami N, et al. Anti-inflammatory effect on colitis and modulation of microbiota by fermented plant extract supplementation. Fermentation. 2021;**7**(55):fermentation7020055

[64] Nomura K, Ishikawa D, Okahara K, Ito S, Haga K, Takahashi M, et al. Bacteroidetes species are correlated with disease activity in ulcerative colitis. Journal of Clinical Medicine. 2021;**10**(8):1749. DOI: 10.3390/jcm10081749

[65] Agista AZ, Rusbana TB, Islam J, Ohsaki Y, Sultana H, Hirakawa R, et al. Fermented Rice bran supplementation prevents the development of intestinal fibrosis due to DSS-induced inflammation in mice. Nutrients. 2021;**13**(6):1869. DOI: 10.3390/nu13061869

[66] Islam J, Koseki T, Watanabe K, Budijanto S, Oikawa A, Alauddin M, et al. Dietary supplementation of fermented rice bran effectively alleviates dextran sodium sulfate-induced colitis in mice. Nutrients. 2017;**9**(7):747. DOI: 10.3390/nu9070747

[67] Li Z, Lu J, Yang Z, Han L, Tan T. Utilization of white rice bran for production of l-lactic acid. Biomass and Bioenergy. 2012;**39**:53-58

[68] Gao MT, Kaneko M, Hirata M, Toorisaka E, Hano T. Utilization of rice bran as nutrient source for fermentative lactic acid production. Bioresource Technology. 2008;**99**(9):3659-3664

[69] Tanaka T, Hoshina M, Tanabe S, Sakai K, Ohtsubo S, Taniguchi M. Production of D-lactic acid from defatted rice bran by simultaneous saccharification and fermentation. Bioresource Technology. 2006;**97**(2):211-217. DOI: 10.1016/j.biortech.2005.02.025

[70] Ali SS, Vidhale NN. Protease production by F usarium o xysporum in solid-state fermentation using rice bran. American Journal of Microbiological Research. 2013;**3**:45-47

[71] Chutmanop J, Chuichulcherm S, Chisti Y, Srinophakun P. Protease production by aspergillus oryzae in solid-state fermentation using agroindustrial substrates. Journal of Chemical Technology and Biotechnology. 2008;**83**:1012-1018

[72] Rajesh MJ, Rajesh L, Abachire LW. Optimization of solid state fermentation conditions for the production of cellulase by using Trichoderma Reesei. European Journal of Applied Engineering and Scientific Research. 2012;**1**(4):196-200

[73] Grover A, Maninder A, Sarao LK. Production of fungal amylase and cellulase enzymes via solid state fermentation using aspergillus Oryzae and Trichoderma Reesei. International Journal of Advancements in Research & Technology. 2013;**2**(8):108-124

[74] Saykhedkar SS, Singhal RS. Solid-state fermentation for production of griseofulvin on rice bran using Penicillium griseofulvum. Biotechnology Progress. 2004;**20**(4):1280-1284

[75] Oliveira Mdos S, Feddern V, Kupski L, Cipolatti EP, Badiale-Furlong E, de Souza-Soares LA. Changes in lipid, fatty acids and phospholipids composition of whole rice bran after solid-state fungal fermentation. Bioresource Technology. 2011;**102**(17):8335-8338. DOI: 10.1016/j.biortech.2011.06.025

[76] Schmidt CG, Gonçalves LM, Prietto L, Hackbart HS, Furlong EB. Antioxidant activity and enzyme inhibition of phenolic acids from fermented rice bran with fungus Rizhopus oryzae. Food Chemistry. 2014;**146**:371-377. DOI: 10.1016/j.foodchem.2013.09.101

Section 6

Interventional IBD in Ulcerative Colitis

Chapter 9

Role of Interventional IBD in Management of Ulcerative Colitis(UC)-Associated Neoplasia and Post-Operative Pouch Complications in UC: A Systematic Review

Partha Pal, Rupa Banerjee, Mohan Ramchandani, Zaheer Nabi, Duvvuru Nageshwar Reddy and Manu Tandan

Abstract

Interventional inflammatory bowel disease (IIBD) is going to play a major role in complex IBD including ulcerative-colitis associated neoplasia (UCAN) and postoperative complications after ileal pouch-anal anastomosis (IPAA) in ulcerative colitis (UC). We performed a literature search in PubMed using keywords such as "UCAN" and "endoscopic management of pouch complications," After screening 1221 citations, finally, 91 relevant citations were identified for the systematic review. Endoscopic recognition of dysplasia should be done by high-definition white light endoscopy (HD-WLE) or dye-based/virtual chromoendoscopy (CE) especially in known dysplasia or primary sclerosing cholangitis (PSC). Endoscopically visible lesions without deep submucosal invasion can be resected endoscopically with endoscopic mucosal resection (EMR), endoscopic submucosal dissection (ESD), or using full-thickness resection device (FTRD). Image-enhanced endoscopy (IEE) and IIBD have an emerging role in screening, diagnosis, and management of colitis-associated neoplasia in UC and can avoid colectomy. IIBD can manage a significant proportion of post-IPAA complications. Pouch strictures can be treated with endoscopic balloon dilation (EBD) or stricturotomy, whereas acute and chronic anastomotic leak or sinuses can be managed with through the scope (TTS)/over the scope clips (OTSC) and endoscopic fistulotomy/sinusotomy.

Keywords: ulcerative colitis-associated neoplasia, Ileal pouch-anal anastomosis, interventional inflammatory bowel disease, ulcerative colitis, pouch complications

1. Introduction

With growing multidisciplinary care model of inflammatory bowel disease (IBD), IIBD is going to play a major role in management of complex IBD. Apart from its major role in management of Crohn's disease-related strictures and fistulas, IIBD has an important role to play in management of colitis-associated neoplasia in ulcerative colitis (UC) and postoperative pouch complications [1, 2]. Ulcerative-colitis associated neoplasia (UCAN) can range from indefinite dysplasia (IND), low-grade dysplasia (LGD), high-grade dysplasia (HGD), invisible dysplasia, and colorectal cancer (CRC). Apart from conventional dysplastic lesions, non-conventional dysplasia (e.g., serrated epithelial change: SEC) can occur in one third. Non-conventional dysplasia increases risk of advanced colorectal neoplasia (aCRN) according to recent meta-analysis and may warrant frequent surveillance [3].

Endoscopic screening should begin at 8–10 years from symptom onset for UCAN in the absence of PSC with subsequent surveillance based on risk stratification. HD-WLE, narrow band imaging (NBI), and CE have similar efficacy in detecting UCAN [4]. The incremental benefit of newer modalities of IEE such as Fuji Intelligent Color Enhancement (FICE), I-SCAN, linked color imaging (LCI), and autofluorescence imaging (AFI) for diagnosis of UCAN compared to conventional screening needs further evaluation. Endocytoscopy and probe-based confocal laser endomicroscopy (pCLE) can be helpful in "in vivo" diagnosis of UCAN [5]. Visible, uni-focal, polypoidal dysplasia of any grade can be resected en bloc using EMR or ESD [6]. For invisible dysplasia, management is dependent on patient-related (e.g., PSC) and histologic factors and includes colectomy. Concurrent inlet strictures in pre-pouch ileitis and anastomotic strictures can be treated with endoscopic balloon dilation or stricturotomy. Stricturing/fistulizing complications of Crohn's disease of the pouch can also be treated endoscopically. Endoscopic sinusotomy and fistulotomy are helpful in treating pouch sinus and fistulas respectively. Endoscopic placement of clips is useful in controlling leaks from pouch. Endoscopic resection can be done for large symptomatic inflammatory polyps in the pouch or polyps in the rectal cuff [2, 7]. We aimed to systematically review all the relevant literature pertaining to endoscopic management of UCAN and pouch complications post IPAA.

2. Search strategy

For the purpose of the review, we searched the PubMed using keywords "ulcerative-colitis associated neoplasia (UCAN)" and "endoscopic management of pouch complications" We found 965 citations. We also screened relevant articles with specific searches and selected cross references. Finally, after screening, total of 1238 citations, 91 were identified for the systematic review (**Figure 1**).

3. Detection of UCAN

Among various modalities for detection of dysplasia in IBD (**Table 1**), high-definition white light endoscopy (HD-WLE), narrow-band imaging (NBI), and chromoendoscopy (CE) were similar in efficacy in detecting UCAN with minor differences among them according to network meta-analysis [4]. Standard definition

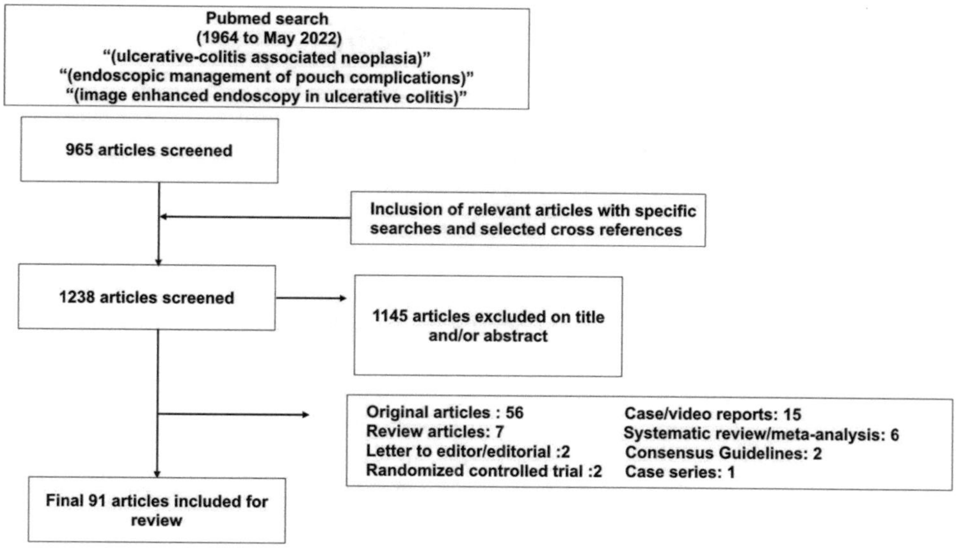

Figure 1.
Consort diagram of systematic review on ulcerative colitis associated neoplasia and post ileal pouch complications.

white light endoscopy (SD- WLE) was shown to be inferior to all these modalities [4]. Shorter withdrawal time and easy applicability are the advantages of NBI compared to CE whereas dysplasia detection rates are similar [8]. Magnifying endoscopy (ME) has incremental benefits over CE for detecting tumor margins to guide endoscopic resection (ER). ME guided ER has R0 resection rate of 95% (compared to 91% with distinct borders with only CE) [9].

The Japanese NBI expert team (JNET) classification and pit pattern on magnifying virtual/chromoendoscopy can predict histological diagnosis and invasion depth accurately as shown in a retrospective study of UCAN who underwent endoscopic resection or colectomy. JNET 2A, 2B, and 3 lesions imply low grade dysplasia (LGD), LGD/high grade dysplasia (HGD), and submucosal invasive carcinoma (SMIC). Pit pattern III/IV, VI low irregularity, VI high irregularity/VN can predict LGD, LGD/HGD, SMIC respectively [10]. Among image-enhanced endoscopy, (IEE), Fuji Intelligent Color Enhancement (FICE) can help predict histology of raised lesions in IBD apart from NBI [11]. I-SCAN is another modality of IEE which has a similar diagnostic yield with a shorter examination time than conventional CE [12]. Linked color imaging (LCI) with indigo carmine dye spraying can help facilitate UCAN diagnosis [13]. Endocytoscopy may help in "in vivo" diagnosis of intra-mucosal carcinoma (IMC) by observing enlarged nuclei after methylene blue staining [14]. Endocytoscopy irregularly-formed nuclei with pit (EC-IN-PIT) guided diagnosis of UCAN were shown to have better specificity and diagnostic accuracy than pit pattern alone in a pilot study [15]. Probe-based confocal laser endomicroscopy (pCLE, Cellvizio, Mauna Kea Technologies, Paris, France) can differentiate UCAN (carcinoma or dysplasia) with accuracy, sensitivity, and specificity of 92%, 100%, and 83%, respectively [16]. Autofluorescence imaging (AFI) can assess the lesion based on fluorescent intensity rather than analysis of surface pattern [17]. AFI with oral 5-aminolevulinic acid sensitization has incremental diagnostic yield compared to WLE [18]. Prospective randomized controlled trial (RCT) did not show any advantage of high definition

Imaging modalities	Potential application in detecting Ulcerative colitis associated neoplasia (UCAN)
High-definition white light endoscopy (HD-WLE)	2-fold better than standard definition white light endoscopy (WLE) in detection of neoplasia on targeted biospy
Dye Chromoendoscopy (DCE)	3.2-fold increase in number of detected intraepithelial neoplasia compared to WLE guided random biopsies, 57.4% incremental yield compared to WLE
Virtual chromoendoscopy	
Narrow band imaging (NBI)	The diagnostic yield is not increased compared to DCE, but shorter withdrawal time and easy applicability are the advantages
Linked color imaging (LCI)	Study in IBD is scanty and limited to case reports
Blue laser imaging	
Dyeless chromoendoscopy	
Fuji Intelligent Color Enhancement	FICE can predict histology of polypoid and non-polypoidal raised lesions based on Kudo's classification and presence of fibrin cap
Autofluorescence imaging	AFI can have incremental diagnostic benefit over WLE based on fluorescent intensity
i-SCAN-OE (Pentax)	Similar diagnostic yield with shorter examination time than conventional CE, combined digital and optical enhancement (OE)
Newer techniques	
Endocytoscopy	It can help "in vivo" diagnosis of intra-mucosal carcinoma (IMC) by observing enlarged nuclei after methylene blue staining. Endocytoscopy irregularly-formed nuclei with pit (EC-IN-PIT) guided diagnosis of neoplasia can have better diagnostic accuracy than pit pattern alone
Probe based confocal laser endomicroscopy	Highly accurate but inflammation and hyperplasia can reduce sensitivity, use of molecular imaging with confocal probes can help in early diagnosis of neoplasia part from predicting response to biologics

Table 1.
Potential applications of various endoscopic imaging modalities in detection of ulcerative colitis associated neoplasia.

chromoendoscopy (HDCE) guided targeted biopsy over HD-WLE guided random biopsies [19]. However, targeted biopsy may be cost-effective and time-saving [20]. An inter-observer agreement study has shown poor agreement on intention to biopsy among endoscopists in non-pedunculated potentially dysplastic lesions in UC [21]. Apart from IEE, EUS-guided assessment of depth of invasion can help in treatment selection [22].

4. Dysplasia in ulcerative colitis and risk of advanced colorectal neoplasia (aCRN)

4.1 Low grade dysplasia

Recurrent low-grade dysplasia (LGD) at first follow-up colonoscopy is a risk factor for aCRN as shown in a population-based registry from Netherlands with a hazard ratio of 1.66. A recurrence-free interval of three years predicts lower probability of subsequent occurrence of aCRN [23]. The risk of progression to aCRN is

0.8% per year. Multifocal LGD, PSC, location in distal colon, and invisible uni-focal low-grade dysplasia are associated with disease progression and hence require colectomy [24]. However, this is not commonly practiced by clinicians with limited experience in surveillance colonoscopy and from non-academic centers [25]. A web-based prediction tool for progression of LGD to aCRN has been recently developed and validated based on these four parameters: endoscopically visible LGD >1 cm, unresectable/incomplete endoscopic resection, moderate/severe histologic inflammation within 5 years of LGD and multifocal LGD [26]. LGD in a case of primary sclerosing cholangitis (PSC) warrants colectomy as the risk of aCRN is considerably high after diagnosis of LGD in PSC (8.4 per patient-years) as compared to LGD in non-PSC patients (3.1 per patient-years). PSC is an independent risk factor for aCRN warranting annual colonoscopic surveillance [27]. Biopsy sampling of surrounding mucosa has limited yield in predicting risk of aCRN whereas the grade of dysplasia predicts aCRN [28].

4.2 Indefinite dysplasia

Indefinite dysplasia (IND) found in nearly 4% of patients can increase the risk of aCRN (3.1% per patient-years) by 6.9-fold after adjusting for other confounding factors [29]. On the other hand, post inflammatory polyps (PIP)/pseudo-polyps were predictive of higher severity of colonic inflammation and colectomy but not aCRN [30].

4.3 Colonic strictures in UC

Colonic stricture in ulcerative colitis was thought to be associated with neoplasia unless proven otherwise. However, strictures may represent inflammatory sequelae as well. Colonic strictures in long-standing colitis do not independently predict advanced colorectal neoplasia as shown in a retrospective cohort study mainly involving Crohn's colitis [31]. Prospective studies in ulcerative colitis-associated strictures are needed to confirm the finding. Non-passable strictures <4/5 cm on computed tomography (CT)-colonography without any evidence of dysplasia on endoscopic biopsy are candidates for endoscopic dilation [32].

4.4 Non-conventional and invisible dysplasia

A study retrospectively evaluating colonoscopic images recorded within last two years prior to diagnosis of UCAN has shown that the mean diagnostic delay for UCAN was nearly 15 months. Visible lesions were present in 25.9%, 18.2%, and 31.3% of UCAN, early- and late-stage cancers, respectively. Invisible lesions were more common in left colon and rectum and was associated with inflammation. UCAN with indistinct margins were more likely to be associated with inflammation than those with distance margins [33]. Two third of the non-conventional dysplasia in IBD (hypermucinous, goblet cell deficient and crypt cell dysplasia) can present with flat/invisible dysplasia (crypt cell:96%, goblet cell deficient-65%, hypermucinous-42%) with equally high risk of subsequent aCRN (HGD or adenocarcinoma: 37% and 23% respectively in those with follow up colonoscopy; goblet cell>hypermucinous>crypt cell) [34]. These findings highlight the need for random biopsies in addition to targeted biopsies as non-conventional dysplasia often co-exist with the conventional dysplasia and can be the only form of dysplasia present. One-fifth of the dysplasias in IBD patients are found on random biopsies [35].

A recent study has highlighted that demarcated red-colored areas histologically characterized by increased vessel density and size (CD 34 positive) can be useful in identifying flat type dysplasia. These areas are common in base of LGD and throughout entire surface of HGD. Targeted biopsy from these areas should be considered [36]. In addition to Kudo's neoplastic pit patterns (III-V), pine-cone/villi pattern on surface morphology are highly specific for neoplasia and hence should be subjected to targeted biopsy [37]. Red in blue sign, pale-whitish mucosa, velvety appearance, ulceration, wall deformity, spontaneous friability and interruption of innominate grooves are signs of non-polypoidal UCAN [38].

4.5 CRN in rectal stump post colectomy in UC

Risk of CRN in rectal stump after ileorectal anastomosis (IRA) post-colectomy in UC is 7.1% and 14% after 10 and 20 years respectively. PSC, age at the time of IRA, UC disease duration and history of colorectal cancer are risk factors of CRN and rectal carcinoma after IRA. Hence ileal pouch anal anastomosis (IPAA) should be considered instead of IRA in high-risk patients such as PSC [39]. Acute severe UC decreases risk of IRA failure whereas Pre-colectomy thiopurine use within 12 months does not increase risk of CRN after IPAA in UC or indeterminate colitis [40].

5. Endoscopic resection of UCAN

(**Figure 2**)

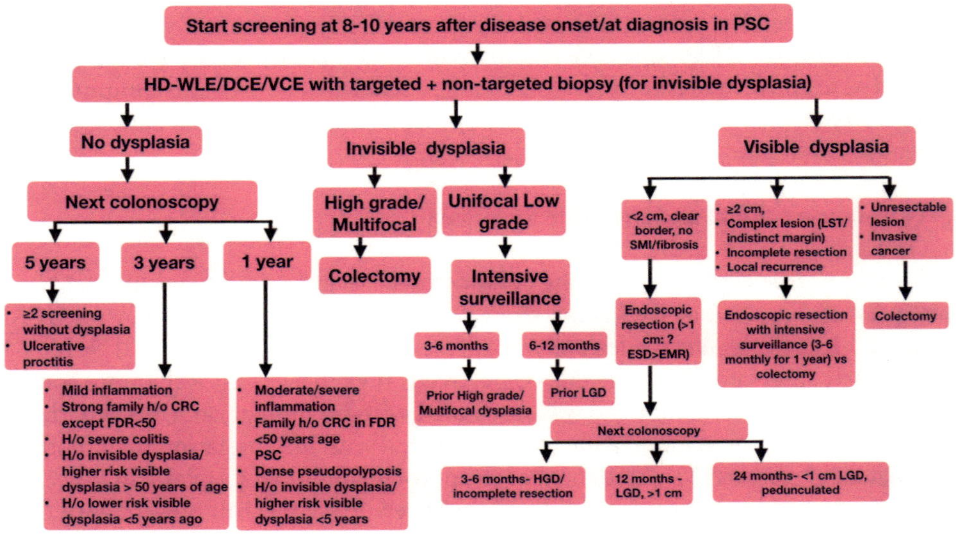

Figure 2.
Algorithm for surveillance and management of ulcerative colitis associated neoplasia. HD-WLE- high-definition white light endoscopy, DCE- dye chromoendoscopy, VCE- virtual chromoendoscopy, CRC- colorectal cancer, FDR- first degree relative, H/o - history of, HGD- high grade dysplasia, LGD- low grade dysplasia, LST- laterally spreading tumor.

5.1 Endoscopic mucosal resection

Earlier colectomy was indicated for any grade of dysplasia until it was recognized that endoscopy resection for polypoidal HGD or endoscopically visible dysplasia (earlier known as dysplasia-associated lesion or mass: DALM) with surveillance can avoid colectomy [41–44]. For polypoidal lesions, there was no difference between outcomes with polypectomy versus proctocolectomy. However, continued close surveillance is mandatory to identify metachronous lesions [45] Similarly it was realized that flat dysplasias can be managed safely with endoscopic mucosal resection (EMR) (**Figure 3** A-D)) [46]. Underwater EMR can be particularly beneficial in resecting UCAN compared to conventional EMR in areas of scarring and severe submucosal fibrosis (SMF) hindering lifting of the lesion [47]. UEMR is safe, effective and time-saving which have shown to remove large polyps in UC with submucosal fibrosis by "heat-sink" and "floating" effects (**Figure 3** E-F) [48].

5.2 Endoscopic submucosal dissection (ESD)

For CAN, the en-bloc and Ro resection rates with ESD are 83% and 67%, respectively. However, a study reported that upto 70% can develop metachronous UCAN on long term follow up which may require colectomy or re-ESD according to a small study [49]. The advantage of ESD is total excision biopsy to evaluate the lesion. Compared to non-UC patients, ESD in UC is associated with lower rate of Ro resection (71% vs. 93%) with lower probability of negative horizontal margin [50]. Hence the demarcation line should be ascertained. Technical difficulties can occur due to scarring and excessive submucosal fibrosis (SMF) which can occur in nearly 40% of cases undergoing ESD [51]. Submucosal fatty infiltration is another limiting factor

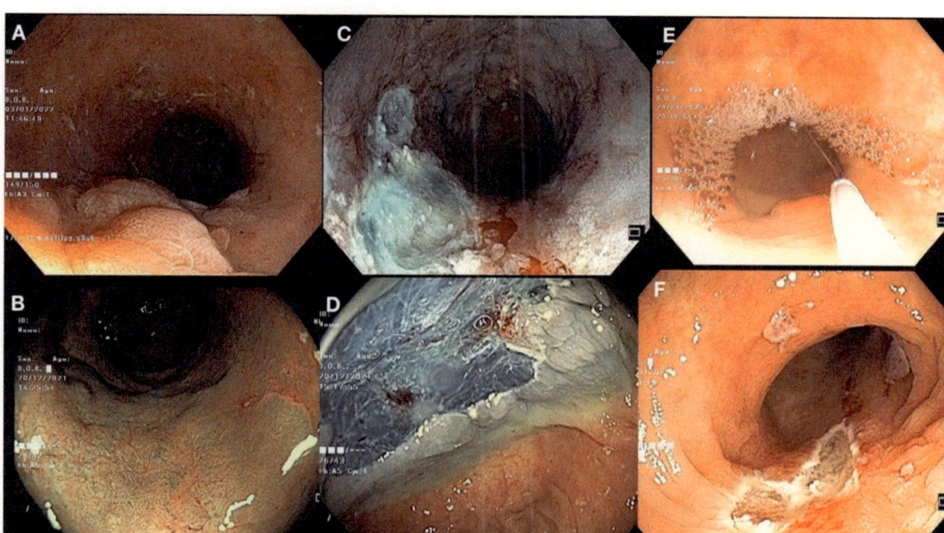

Figure 3.
Endoscopic mucosal resection (EMR) for ulcerative colitis associated neoplasia. A, B- flat visible dysplasias in a case of long-standing ulcerative colitis, C, D- EMR site post resection- biopsy showed high grade dysplasia, D, E- underwater EMR done for residual neoplasia post initial session of EMR.

for ESD in UCAN [52]. Analysis of colectomy specimens have shown that 21% of the lesions can be invisible endoscopically highlighting the importance of intensive surveillance colonoscopy [51]. To overcome the effect of SMF, multi-traction technique using three intertwined loops with clips have been used to treat recurrence of HGD in UC [53]. Another study in 133 colorectal neoplasms (28 with UC) with submucosal fibrosis (28 had UC) water pressure assisted ESD (WP-ESD) had significantly shorter procedure time related to conventional ESD [54].

In a meta-analysis of 203 dysplastic lesions (mean size 2.7 cm, 83% left colon, 90% non-polypoid,) in 192 UC patients, the en bloc resection, complete resection, and R0 resection rates were 94%, 84%, and 81% respectively. SMF was seen in 71%. Mean procedure time was 83 minutes. The rates of local recurrence, metachronous tumor and additional surgery were 5%, 6%, and 10% respectively. Adverse events like bleeding and perforation were seen in 8% and 6%, respectively [55]. Another systematic review showed comparable en bloc and R0 resection rates (88.4% and 78.2% respectively) [56]. Results of ESD in UCAN is best for those with non-invasive pit/vascular pattern, no surface ulceration, distinct borders and appropriate lifting on submucosal injection [57]. Results of ESD for non-polypoidal UCAN is inferior to those for polypoidal lesions due to SMF in 90–100% patients: en-bloc and curative resection rates are 60–100% and 70–79% respectively. Adverse events and recurrence occurred in <10% and 4–20% respectively [58–60].

Prior to widespread use of ESD, endoscopic piecemeal resection followed by argon plasma coagulation had been described in the past for large, poorly lifting adenomas [61].

5.3 Choice of an endoscopic resection technique in UCAN

The choice between ESD and EMR for UCAN can be decided based on a recent study which showed that ESD has higher R0 resection rates than EMR for ≥11 mm lesions (94% vs. 55%) and non-polypoidal lesions (100% vs. 55%). Hence it was concluded that EMR can be preferred for lesions ≤10 mm. 10% patients had intra-procedure perforation during ESD and metachronous HGD noted in 3% [62]. Another study concluded that EMR is indicated for small lesions without fibrosis and ESD for large lesions with fibrosis [63]. Overall, it is important to note that endoscopic resection techniques can help in preventing colectomy by removal of large CRNs [64].

5.4 Modalities other than EMR or ESD

Hybrid resection with ESD and FTRD can be useful in lesions with severe submucosal fibrosis. Hybrid ESD can be useful in large laterally spreading tumor [65]. ESD assisted EMR had been described as early as in 2008 in a series of 67 patients, which reported en-bloc resection rate of 78% with R0 resection rate of 94% in those undergoing en-bloc resection [66]. A recent report first described use of FTRD in a case of long-standing UC for a non-lifting, fibrotic adenoma in descending colon [67].

5.5 Risk of recurrence

The chance of recurrence of cancer and any dysplasia after endoscopic resection of polypoid dysplasia in UC are 5.3 cases/1000 patient-years and 65 cases/1000 patient-years, respectively [68].

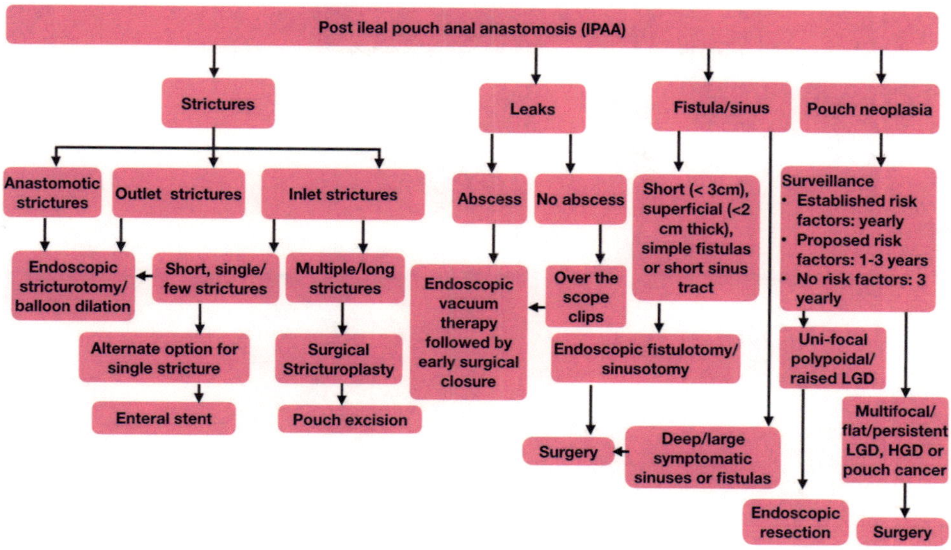

Figure 4.
Management algorithm for endoscopic management of complications after ileal pouch anal anastomosis. HGD- high grade dysplasia, LGD- low grade dysplasia.

6. Role of IIBD in postoperative pouch complications in UC

Among pouch related complications, pouch strictures, floppy pouch complex, acute and chronic anastomotic leak or sinuses can be amenable to endoscopic therapy (**Figure 4**) [69].

6.1 Pouch strictures

Pouch outlet stricture related to sealed ileal pouch have been treated with wire guided stricturotomy using insulated tip (IT) knife [70]. Pouch strictures (inlet and outlet) can be successfully dilated with controlled radial expansion (CRE) balloon relieving symptoms, restoring pouch patency and improved quality of life in a study by Shen et al. of 19 patients with pouch strictures (11 had Crohn's disease of the pouch) [71]. The clinical success of endoscopic balloon dilation (EBD) is 66.7% as reported in a study by Kirat et al. with rest requiring excision of pouch. Nearly half require repeat EBD. Pouch inlet/afferent limb strictures can be treated effectively with both EBD and endoscopic stricturotomy (ES) with comparable surgery free survival as shown by Lan et al. (160 EBD, 40 EST) [72]. The risk of bleeding is higher with ES (4.7% vs. 0% with EBD) whereas the risk of perforation is higher with EBD (0.8% vs. 0% with ES). Length of stricture (>5 cm) and pouchitis are predictors of subsequent surgery [72]. Another study reporting 88 dilations in 20 patients (majority 87% had ileo-anal anastomotic strictures, 95% had UC) showed a technical and clinical success of EBD as 98% and 95% respectively without any major adverse events. The study hence concluded that EBD should be the first line for pouch strictures [73]. In the largest study of 150 patients undergoing 646 EBD procedures, perforations and bleeding occurred in less than 1% cases. At a median follow up of nearly 10 years, 87.3% retained their pouches. Multiple strictures and Crohn's disease of the pouch were independent predictors of pouch failure [74].

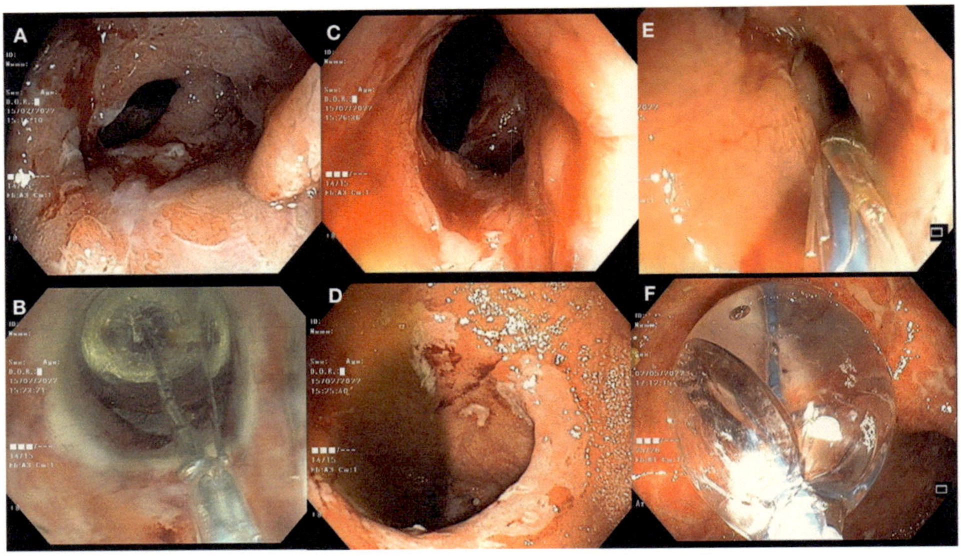

Figure 5.
Endoscopic management of pouch strictures. A. Ileal pouch anastomotic stricture, B. endoscopic balloon dilation (EBD) being performed, C. stricture post EBD, D. Pouchitis noted in ileal pouch post anastomotic dilation, E. pouch inlet stricture, F. EBD for pouch inlet stricture.

Based on results of various studies, a systematic review has concluded that for pouch anal strictures, bougie dilation followed by balloon dilation (**Figure 5** A-D) are the modalities prior to surgical dilation. Endocarp guided needle knife stricturotomy is another alternative approach [75]. Pouch inlet strictures need to be treated with both medical (for inflammatory stricture) and endoscopic therapy (EBD) (for fibrotic stricture) (Figure E-F) [75]. Mid pouch stricture has been treated with surgical stricturoplasty rather than excision of pouch [75].

6.2 Pouch leaks

Successful management of leak from the "tip of the J" have been described with two over the scope clips (OTSCs) [76]. OTSCs have been shown to be successful in nearly two thirds of the patients with one or two sessions in closing such leaks while remaining require revision surgery. 50% patients required re-procedure (OTSC clip or endoscopic suturing) and finally one third required surgery [77]. Apart from direct closure of defects, a short period of endoscopic vacuum therapy (EVT) with periodic sponge changes can help in early surgical closure for treating anastomotic leakage post IPAA. 100% secondary anastomotic healing (median healing time 48 days) was achieved in early closure group (n = 15) compared to 52% (median healing time 70 days) in conventional treatment group (n = 29) [78]. In another series of 8 patients, complete healing of leak was documented in median 2 months-time [79]. Hence EVT can be used for anastomotic leak post IPAA whereas OTSC is to be used if there is leak without any abscess [7].

6.3 Pouch fistula

Endoscopic fistulotomy can be used in short (< 3 cm), superficial (<2 cm thick), simple fistulas like pouch-to-pouch body fistula, perianal fistula and ileo-cecal fistula

[7]. In a study of 29 patients (26 IPAA, 21 having UC) with IBD related fistulas, endoscopic fistulotomy (EFT) with needle knife was successful in healing fistula in nearly 90% patients whereas 10% require surgical intervention [80]. Preliminary results of another study comparing EFT with redo-surgery showed complete healing in all cases of redo surgery with complete and partial fistula healing in 78.4% and 21.6% wire EFT respectively. Rate of subsequent surgery and adverse events were lower in EFT arm (n = 40) compared to redo surgery (n = 19) [81]. Combined use of multiple sessions of endoscopic clipping and EFT have been used to completely heal pouch-to-pouch fistula from tip of the "J" to the anastomosis [82].

6.4 Pouch sinus

Endoscopic sinusotomy can be successfully used to manage chronic pouch anastomotic sinus after IPAA in UC with fair healing rate (53.2% complete, 15.3% partial) as compared to 94% initial complete healing rate with redo surgery as shown in a historical cohort study (endoscopic sinusotomy 141, surgery 85). However, redo surgery was associated with higher morbidity (43.5%) vs. compared to endoscopic sinusotomy (2.5%). Subsequent recurrence and need for surgery were not significantly higher in endoscopic arm as compared to surgical closure [83]. Like pouch fistulas, EVT can be helpful in treating anastomotic leak post IPAA preventing development of chronic pre-sacral sinus [84]. Multiple sessions of endoscopic sinusotomy under doppler ultrasound guidance have been used along with topical doxycycline (100 mg IV with 10 ml saline) (a matrix metalloproteinase inhibitor which promote fibrosis) injection for refractory sinus post IPAA [85]. However, endoscopic therapy is reserved for small sinus tracts whereas surgery may be required for large, deep symptomatic sinuses [86].

Few studies have evaluated factors influencing sinus healing and pouch survival with endoscopic sinusotomy. Crohn's disease of the pouch is a negative predictor of pouch healing whereas higher BMI and longer intervals between sinusotomy were positive predictors [87]. Conversely, another study by the same group have shown that excess BMI gain (≥ 10%) post sinusotomy was associated with recurrent sinus [88]. With regard to surgery free survival, acute anastomotic leak, toxic megacolon, longer sinus and delayed sinusotomy were risk factors; whereas longer interval between sinusotomies, concurrent 50% dextrose and doxycycline use were protective factors [87]. Endoscopic hemostasis for severe bleeding in diverted ileal pouch have been described with spray of hypertonic saline (50% dextrose) [89]. Incremental number of endoscopic sinusotomy increase the chances of sinus healing whereas delay in sinus diagnosis and complex sinuses are negative predictors of success as shown in another study of 65 patients [90].

6.5 Floppy pouch complex

Floppy pouch complex is managed initially with lifestyle modifications like avoidance of excessive straining failing which endoscopic ligation/plication can be considered [69].

6.6 Pouch neoplasia

Low grade dysplasia, high grade dysplasia, adenocarcinomas and squamous cell carcinomas are reported to occur in pouch after IPAA. Presence of established (pre-colectomy cancer or dysplasia) and proposed risk factors (PSC, family history of colon cancer, chronic pouch inflammation, long standing UC, type "C" mucosa- atrophic mucosa with chronic inflammation) predict risk of pouch neoplasia and direct pouch surveillance [91]. Presence of established risk factors warrant annual surveillance pouchoscopy with at least 3 biopsies from cuff/anal transition zone, pouch inlet and body or any endoscopically visible lesion [2]. Presence of proposed risk factors warrant pouchoscopy with biopsy every 1–3 years. Surveillance pouchoscopy is recommended every 3 years in patients without risk factors [2]. Surveillance is important given the fact that pouch neoplasia has poor prognosis and early detection can salvage pouch. After endoscopic resection of uni-focal polypoidal/raised LGD by polypectomy/EMR/ESD, surveillance should be done every 3 months for 2 years. Irrespective of the modality of endoscopic resection (EMR/ESD), the resection should be en-bloc with extensive biopsy of adjacent mucosa. Multifocal/flat/persistent LGD, HGD or pouch cancer should be treated with surgical intervention (excision, mucosectomy or pouch advancement). People with established risk factors of pouch neoplasia may require complete proctectomy [91] .

7. Conclusion

The role of interventional endoscopy in diagnosis and management of ulcerative colitis associated neoplasia and pouch complications post colectomy in UC are expanding. While HD-WLE and CE are established methods of screening for UCAN, other modalities of virtual CE are emerging. Endocytoscopy and pCLE have the potential for "in vivo" diagnosis of dysplasia. EMR, ESD and recently FTRD have been employed for endoscopic resection of UCAN. Underwater EMR and traction or water pressure assisted ESD can help in resecting UCAN in the presence of submucosal fibrosis. Among pouch related complications, pouch strictures, leaks, fistula, sinus, pouch neoplasia and floppy pouch can be managed endoscopically. Future prospective and comparative studies are required to further define the role of IIBD in the current management algorithm of UCAN and pouch complications.

Authors' contribution

Concept and design: PP; **Administrative support:** MT, DNR; **Provision of study material/patients:** PP; **Acquisition of data:** PP. **Data Analysis and interpretation:** PP; **Preparation of initial draft:** PP,; **Critical revision of the manuscript:** MT, RB, DNR, **Important intellectual inputs and revision:** MT, RB, ZN, MR, DNR **Manuscript writing:** All authors, **Approval of final manuscript:** All authors.

Author details

Partha Pal*, Rupa Banerjee, Mohan Ramchandani, Zaheer Nabi,
Duvvuru Nageshwar Reddy and Manu Tandan
Department of Medical Gastroenterology, Asian Institute of Gastroenterology,
Hyderabad, Telangana, India

*Address all correspondence to: partha0123456789@gmail.com

References

[1] Shen B, Kochhar G, Navaneethan U, Farraye FA, Schwartz DA, Iacucci M, et al. Practical guidelines on endoscopic treatment for Crohn's disease strictures: A consensus statement from the global interventional inflammatory bowel disease group. The Lancet Gastroenterology & Hepatology. 2020;**5**(4):393-405

[2] Shen B, Kochhar GS, Kariv R, Liu X, Navaneethan U, Rubin DT, et al. Diagnosis and classification of ileal pouch disorders: Consensus guidelines from the international Ileal pouch consortium. The Lancet Gastroenterology & Hepatology. 2021;**6**(10):826-849

[3] Parian AM, Limketkai BN, Chowdhury R, Brewer GG, Salem G, Falloon K, et al. Serrated epithelial change is associated with high rates of neoplasia in ulcerative colitis patients: A case-controlled study and systematic review with meta-analysis. Inflammatory Bowel Diseases. 2021;**27**(9):1475-1481

[4] Gondal B, Haider H, Komaki Y, Komaki F, Micic D, Rubin DT, et al. Efficacy of various endoscopic modalities in detecting dysplasia in ulcerative colitis: A systematic review and network meta-analysis. World Journal of Gastrointestinal Endoscopy. 2020;**12**(5):159-171

[5] Iacucci M, Furfaro F, Matsumoto T, Uraoka T, Smith S, Ghosh S, et al. Advanced endoscopic techniques in the assessment of inflammatory bowel disease: New technology, new era. Gut. 2019;**68**(3):562-572

[6] Axelrad JE, Shah SC. Diagnosis and management of inflammatory bowel disease-associated neoplasia: Considerations in the modern era. Therapeutic Advances in Gastroenterology. 2020;**13**:1756284820920779

[7] Chandan S, Shen B, Kochhar GS. Therapeutic endoscopy in postoperative pouch complications. Clinics in Colon and Rectal Surgery. 2022;**35**(1):78-88

[8] Bisschops R, Bessissow T, Joseph JA, Baert F, Ferrante M, Ballet V, et al. Chromoendoscopy versus narrow band imaging in UC: A prospective randomised controlled trial. Gut. 2018;**67**(6):1087-1094

[9] Nishio M, Hirasawa K, Ozeki Y, Sawada A, Ikeda R, Fukuchi T, et al. Magnifying endoscopy is useful for tumor border diagnosis in ulcerative colitis patients. Digestive and Liver Disease. Jun 2022;**54**(6):812-818

[10] Kawasaki K, Nakamura S, Esaki M, Kurahara K, Eizuka M, Nuki Y, et al. Clinical usefulness of magnifying colonoscopy for the diagnosis of ulcerative colitis-associated neoplasia. Digestive Endoscopy. 2019;**31**(Suppl. 1):36-42

[11] Cassinotti A, Buffoli F, Fociani P, Staiano T, Villanacci V, Nebuloni M, et al. Virtual Chromoendoscopy with FICE for the classification of polypoid and nonpolypoid raised lesions in ulcerative colitis. Journal of Clinical Gastroenterology. 2019;**53**(4):269-276

[12] Lopez-Serrano A, Suarez MJ, Beso P, Algarra A, Latorre P, Barrachina MM, et al. Virtual chromoendoscopy with iSCAN as an alternative method to dye-spray chromoendoscopy for dysplasia detection in long-standing colonic inflammatory bowel disease:

A case-control study. Scandinavian Journal of Gastroenterology. 2021;**56**(7):820-828

[13] Kanmura S, Tanaka A, Komaki Y, Ido A. A case of screening colonoscopy using linked-color imaging to detect ulcerative colitis-associated colorectal cancer. Digestive and Liver Disease. 2019;**51**(7):1061

[14] Misawa M, Kudo SE, Ogata N. Two cases of colitis-associated neoplasia observed with endocytoscopy. Digestive Endoscopy. 2019;**31**(Suppl. 1):43-44

[15] Kudo SE, Maeda Y, Ogata N, Misawa M, Ogawa Y, Takishima K, et al. Combined endocytoscopy with pit pattern diagnosis in ulcerative colitis-associated neoplasia: Pilot study. Digestive Endoscopy. 2022;**34**(1):133-143

[16] Ohmiya N, Horiguchi N, Tahara T, Yoshida D, Yamada H, Nagasaka M, et al. Usefulness of confocal laser endomicroscopy to diagnose ulcerative colitis-associated neoplasia. Digestive Endoscopy. 2017;**29**(5):626-633

[17] Moriichi K, Fujiya M, Okumura T. The efficacy of autofluorescence imaging in the diagnosis of colorectal diseases. Clinical Journal of Gastroenterology. 2016;**9**(4):175-183

[18] Kato T, Iwasaki T, Arihiro S, Saruta M. Endoscopic visualization of cancer and dysplasia in patients with ulcerative colitis following sensitization with oral 5-aminolevulinic acid. Journal of Digestive Diseases. 2020;**21**(9):498-504

[19] Yang DH, Park SJ, Kim HS, Park YS, Park DI, Lee KM, et al. High-definition Chromoendoscopy versus high-definition white light colonoscopy for neoplasia surveillance in ulcerative colitis: A randomized controlled trial. The American Journal of Gastroenterology. 2019;**114**(10):1642-1648

[20] Watanabe T, Ajioka Y, Mitsuyama K, Watanabe K, Hanai H, Nakase H, et al. Comparison of targeted vs random biopsies for surveillance of ulcerative colitis-associated colorectal cancer. Gastroenterology. 2016;**151**(6):1122-1130

[21] Yang DH, John S, Mitsuhiro F, Cha JM, Byeon JS, Kim HW, et al. Endoscopic diagnosis of nonpedunculated dysplasia during surveillance of ulcerative colitis: A survey-based multinational study. Gut Liver. 2020;**14**(5):611-618

[22] Kobayashi K, Kawagishi K, Ooka S, Yokoyama K, Sada M, Koizumi W. Clinical usefulness of endoscopic ultrasonography for the evaluation of ulcerative colitis-associated tumors. World Journal of Gastroenterology. 2015;**21**(9):2693-2699

[23] de Jong ME, Nagtegaal ID, Vos S, van der Post RS, van Herwaarden Y, Derikx LAAP, et al. Increased Colorectal Neoplasia Risk in Patients with Inflammatory Bowel Disease and Serrated Polyps with Dysplasia. Digestive Diseases and Sciences. 5 Apr 2022. DOI: 10.1007/s10620-022-07485-w. Epub ahead of print. PMID: 35380348

[24] Fumery M, Dulai PS, Gupta S, Prokop LJ, Ramamoorthy S, Sandborn WJ, et al. Incidence, risk factors, and outcomes of colorectal cancer in patients with ulcerative colitis with low-grade dysplasia: A systematic review and meta-analysis. Clinical Gastroenterology and Hepatology. 2017;**15**(5):665-74 e5

[25] Kabir M, Thomas-Gibson S, Hart AL, Wilson A. Perception of cancer risk and management practice

for colitis-associated dysplasia is influenced by colonoscopy experience and workplace affiliation: Results of an international clinician survey. Journal of Crohn's & Colitis. 2022;**16**(1):39-48

[26] Curtius K, Kabir M, Al Bakir I, Choi CHR, Hartono JL, Johnson M, et al. Multicentre derivation and validation of a colitis-associated colorectal cancer risk prediction web tool. Gut. 2022;**71**(4):705-715

[27] Shah SC, Ten Hove JR, Castaneda D, Palmela C, Mooiweer E, Colombel JF, et al. High risk of advanced colorectal neoplasia in patients with primary Sclerosing cholangitis associated with inflammatory bowel disease. Clinical Gastroenterology and Hepatology. 2018;**16**(7):1106-13 e3

[28] Krugliak Cleveland N, Torres J, Rubin DT. What does disease progression look like in ulcerative colitis, and how might it Be prevented? Gastroenterology. 2022;**162**(5):1396-1408

[29] Mahmoud R, Shah SC, Torres J, Castaneda D, Glass J, Elman J, et al. Association between indefinite dysplasia and advanced neoplasia in patients with inflammatory bowel diseases undergoing surveillance. Clinical Gastroenterology and Hepatology. 2020;**18**(7):1518-27e3

[30] Mahmoud R, Shah SC, Ten Hove JR, Torres J, Mooiweer E, Castaneda D, et al. No association between Pseudopolyps and colorectal neoplasia in patients with inflammatory bowel diseases. Gastroenterology. 2019;**156**(5):1333-44e3

[31] Axelrad JE, Faye A, Slaughter JC, Harpaz N, Itzkowitz SH, Shah SC. Colorectal Strictures in Patients With Inflammatory Bowel Disease Do Not Independently Predict Colorectal Neoplasia. Inflammatory Bowel Disease. 3 Jun 2022;**28**(6):855-861

[32] Fumery M, Yzet C, Chatelain D, Yzet T, Brazier F, LeMouel JP, et al. Colonic strictures in inflammatory bowel disease: Epidemiology, complications, and management. Journal of Crohn's & Colitis. 2021;**15**(10):1766-1773

[33] Hisabe T, Matsui T, Yamasaki K, Morokuma T, Aomi K, Yoshizawa N, et al. Possible Earlier Diagnosis of Ulcerative Colitis-Associated Neoplasia: A Retrospective Analysis of Interval Cases during Surveillance. Journal of Clinical Medicine. 29 Apr 2021;**10**(9):1927. DOI: 10.3390/jcm10091927. PMID: 33946906; PMCID: PMC8124807

[34] Choi WT, Salomao M, Zhao L, Alpert L, Setia N, Liao X, et al. Hypermucinous, goblet cell-deficient and crypt cell Dysplasias in inflammatory bowel disease are often associated with flat/invisible endoscopic appearance and advanced neoplasia on follow-up. Journal of Crohn's & Colitis. 2022;**16**(1):98-108

[35] Hu AB, Burke KE, Kochar B, Ananthakrishnan AN. Yield of random biopsies during colonoscopies in inflammatory bowel disease patients undergoing dysplasia surveillance. Inflammatory Bowel Diseases. 2021;**27**(6):779-786

[36] Ikebata A, Shimoda M, Okabayashi K, Uraoka T, Maehata T, Sugimoto S, et al. Demarcated redness associated with increased vascular density/size: A useful marker of flat-type dysplasia in patients with ulcerative colitis. Endoscopy International Open. 2021;**9**(4):E552-Ee61

[37] Shinagawa T, Hata K, Morikawa T, Takiyama H, Emoto S, Murono K, et al. Pine-cone and villi patterns are endoscopic signs suggestive of ulcerative colitis-associated colorectal cancer and dysplasia. Gastrointestinal Endoscopy. 2019;**89**(3):565-75e3

[38] Soetikno R, East J, Suzuki N, Uedo N, Matsumoto T, Watanabe K, et al. Endoscopic submucosal dissection for nonpolypoid colorectal dysplasia in patients with inflammatory bowel disease: in medias res. Gastrointestinal Endoscopy. 2018;**87**(4):1085-1094

[39] Uzzan M, Kirchgesner J, Oubaya N, Amiot A, Gornet JM, Seksik P, et al. Risk of rectal neoplasia after colectomy and Ileorectal anastomosis for ulcerative colitis. Journal of Crohn's & Colitis. 2017;**11**(8):930-935

[40] Kayal M, Riggs A, Plietz M, Khaitov S, Sylla P, Greenstein AJ, et al. The association between pre-colectomy thiopurine use and risk of neoplasia after ileal pouch anal anastomosis in patients with ulcerative colitis or indeterminate colitis: A propensity score analysis. International Journal of Colorectal Disease. 2022;**37**(1):123-130

[41] Engelsgjerd M, Farraye FA, Odze RD. Polypectomy may be adequate treatment for adenoma-like dysplastic lesions in chronic ulcerative colitis. Gastroenterology. 1999;**117**(6):1288-1294 discussion 488-91

[42] Rubin PH, Friedman S, Harpaz N, Goldstein E, Weiser J, Schiller J, et al. Colonoscopic polypectomy in chronic colitis: Conservative management after endoscopic resection of dysplastic polyps. Gastroenterology. 1999;**117**(6):1295-1300

[43] Gorfine SR, Bauer JJ, Harris MT, Kreel I. Dysplasia complicating chronic ulcerative colitis: Is immediate colectomy warranted? Diseases of the Colon and Rectum. 2000;**43**(11):1575-1581

[44] Blonski W, Kundu R, Furth EF, Lewis J, Aberra F, Lichtenstein GR. High-grade dysplastic adenoma-like mass lesions are not an indication for colectomy in patients with ulcerative colitis. Scandinavian Journal of Gastroenterology. 2008;**43**(7):817-820

[45] Vieth M, Behrens H, Stolte M. Sporadic adenoma in ulcerative colitis: Endoscopic resection is an adequate treatment. Gut. 2006;**55**(8):1151-1155

[46] Hurlstone DP, Sanders DS, Atkinson R, Hunter MD, McAlindon ME, Lobo AJ, et al. Endoscopic mucosal resection for flat neoplasia in chronic ulcerative colitis: Can we change the endoscopic management paradigm? Gut. 2007;**56**(6):838-846

[47] Takabayashi K, Kato M, Sasaki M, Iwao Y, Ogata H, Kanai T, et al. Underwater endoscopic mucosal resection for a sporadic adenoma located at severe longitudinal ulcer scars in ulcerative colitis. Endoscopy. 2022;**54**(1):E30-Ee1

[48] Hosotani K, Inoue S, Takahashi K, Hara S, Inokuma T. Underwater endoscopic mucosal resection for complete R0 removal of colorectal polyp in a patient with ulcerative colitis. Endoscopy. 2022;**54**(1):E3-e4

[49] Matsumoto K, Oka S, Tanaka S, Tanaka H, Boda K, Yamashita K, et al. Long-term outcomes after endoscopic submucosal dissection for ulcerative colitis-associated dysplasia. Digestion. 2021;**102**(2):205-215

[50] Matsui A, Hoteya S, Hayasaka J, Yamashita S, Ochiai Y, Suzuki Y, et al. Real-world experience of endoscopic submucosal dissection for ulcerative colitis-associated neoplasia. Inflammatory Intestinal Diseases. 2021;**6**(2):70-77

[51] Kasuga K, Yamada M, Shida D, Tagawa T, Takamaru H, Sekiguchi M, et al. Treatment outcomes of endoscopic submucosal dissection and surgery for colorectal neoplasms in patients

with ulcerative colitis. United European Gastroenterology Journal. 2021;**9**(8):964-972

[52] Mizuno KI, Yokoyama J, Terai S. Management of endoscopic submucosal dissection for ulcerative colitis-associated neoplasia: Tips and pitfalls. Digestive Endoscopy. 2019;**31**(Suppl. 1):44-45

[53] Yzet C, Lambin T, Lafeuille P, Fumery M, Pofelski J, Cotte E, et al. Endoscopic submucosal dissection of high-grade dysplasia recurrence in ulcerative colitis using a multitraction technique. Endoscopy. Aug 2022;**54**(8): E433-E434. DOI: 10.1055/a-1581-7361. Epub 2021 Sep 8. PMID: 34496442

[54] Ozeki Y, Hirasawa K, Ikeda R, Onodera S, Sawada A, Nishio M, et al. Safety and efficacy of water pressure endoscopic submucosal dissection for colorectal tumors with submucosal fibrosis (with video). Gastrointestinal Endoscopy. 2021;**94**(3):607-17.e2

[55] Zeng QS, Zhao ZJ, Nie J, Zou M, Yang JH, Zhang JZ, et al. Efficacy and safety of endoscopic submucosal dissection for dysplasia in ulcerative colitis patients: A systematic review and meta-analysis. Gastroenterology Research and Practice. 2022;**2022**:9556161

[56] Manta R, Zullo A, Telesca DA, Castellani D, Germani U, Reggiani Bonetti L, et al. Endoscopic submucosal dissection for visible dysplasia treatment in ulcerative colitis patients: Cases series and systematic review of literature. Journal of Crohn's & Colitis. 2021;**15**(1):165-168

[57] Yang DH, Kim J, Song EM, Chang K, Lee SH, Hwang SW, et al. Outcomes of ulcerative colitis-associated dysplasia patients referred for potential endoscopic submucosal dissection. Journal of Gastroenterology and Hepatology. 2019;**34**(9):1581-1589

[58] Iacopini F, Saito Y, Yamada M, Grossi C, Rigato P, Costamagna G, et al. Curative endoscopic submucosal dissection of large nonpolypoid superficial neoplasms in ulcerative colitis (with videos). Gastrointestinal Endoscopy. 2015;**82**(4):734-738

[59] Suzuki N, Toyonaga T, East JE. Endoscopic submucosal dissection of colitis-related dysplasia. Endoscopy. 2017;**49**(12):1237-1242

[60] Kinoshita S, Uraoka T, Nishizawa T, Naganuma M, Iwao Y, Ochiai Y, et al. The role of colorectal endoscopic submucosal dissection in patients with ulcerative colitis. Gastrointestinal Endoscopy. 2018;**87**(4):1079-1084

[61] Matsumura K, Nakase H, Chiba T. Combination of endoscopic resection and heat ablation is a promising endoscopic therapy for adenoma-like dysplastic lesion in chronic ulcerative colitis. Case Reports in Gastroenterology. 2009;**3**(1):121-124

[62] Nishio M, Hirasawa K, Ozeki Y, Sawada A, Ikeda R, Fukuchi T, et al. An endoscopic treatment strategy for superficial tumors in patients with ulcerative colitis. Journal of Gastroenterology and Hepatology. 2021;**36**(2):498-506

[63] Alkandari A, Thayalasekaran S, Bhandari M, Przybysz A, Bugajski M, Bassett P, et al. Endoscopic resections in inflammatory bowel disease: A multicentre European outcomes study. Journal of Crohn's & Colitis. 2019;**13**(11):1394-1400

[64] Lightner AL, Vaidya P, Allende D, Gorgun E. Endoscopic submucosal dissection is safe and feasible, allowing for ongoing surveillance and organ preservation in patients with

inflammatory bowel disease. Colorectal Disease. 2021;**23**(8):2100-2107

[65] Gulati S, Emmanuel A, Burt M, Dubois P, Hayee B, Haji A. Outcomes of endoscopic resections of large laterally spreading colorectal lesions in inflammatory bowel disease: A single United Kingdom center experience. Inflammatory Bowel Diseases. 2018;**24**(6):1196-1203

[66] Smith LA, Baraza W, Tiffin N, Cross SS, Hurlstone DP. Endoscopic resection of adenoma-like mass in chronic ulcerative colitis using a combined endoscopic mucosal resection and cap assisted submucosal dissection technique. Inflammatory Bowel Diseases. 2008;**14**(10):1380-1386

[67] Baker GVJ, Kochhar GS. Endoscopic full-thickness resection for the Management of a Polyp in a patient with ulcerative colitis. Cureus. 2022;**14**(5):e24688

[68] Wanders LK, Dekker E, Pullens B, Bassett P, Travis SP, East JE. Cancer risk after resection of polypoid dysplasia in patients with longstanding ulcerative colitis: A meta-analysis. Clinical Gastroenterology and Hepatology. 2014;**12**(5):756-764

[69] Shen B, Fleshner P, Shah SA. How do I diagnose and manage Ileal pouch disorders? The American Journal of Gastroenterology. 2021;**116**(4):621-624

[70] Khan F, Shen B. Wire-guided stricturotomy for sealed ileal pouch. Endoscopy. 2019;**51**(5):493-494

[71] Shen B, Fazio VW, Remzi FH, Delaney CP, Achkar JP, Bennett A, et al. Endoscopic balloon dilation of ileal pouch strictures. The American Journal of Gastroenterology. 2004;**99**(12):2340-2347

[72] Lan N, Wu JJ, Wu XR, Hull LT, Shen B. Endoscopic treatment of pouch inlet and afferent limb strictures: Stricturotomy vs. balloon dilation. Surgical Endoscopy. 2021;**35**(4):1722-1733

[73] Fumery M, Patel NS, Boland BS, Dulai PS, Singh S, Sandborn WJ. Efficacy and safety of endoscopic balloon dilatation of Ileoanal pouch strictures. Inflammatory Bowel Diseases. 2018;**24**(6):1316-1320

[74] Shen B, Lian L, Kiran RP, Queener E, Lavery IC, Fazio VW, et al. Efficacy and safety of endoscopic treatment of ileal pouch strictures. Inflammatory Bowel Diseases. 2011;**17**(12):2527-2535

[75] Segal JP, Adegbola SO, Worley GHT, Sahnan K, Tozer P, Lung PFC, et al. A systematic review: The management and outcomes of Ileal pouch strictures. Journal of Crohn's & Colitis. 2018;**12**(3):369-375

[76] Lescaille Y, Rosh JR, Kiran RP, Shen B. Successful closure of the tip of the "J" fistula of the Ileal pouch with double over-the-scope clips. ACG Case Reports Journal. 2021;**8**(4):e00566

[77] Kochhar GS, Shen B. Endoscopic treatment of leak at the tip of the "J" ileal pouch. Endoscopy International Open. 2017;**5**(1):E64-Ee6

[78] Gardenbroek TJ, Musters GD, Buskens CJ, Ponsioen CY, D'Haens GR, Dijkgraaf MG, et al. Early reconstruction of the leaking ileal pouch-anal anastomosis: A novel solution to an old problem. Colorectal Disease. 2015;**17**(5):426-432

[79] Rottoli M, Di Simone MP, Vallicelli C, Vittori L, Liguori G, Boschi L, et al. Endoluminal vacuum-assisted therapy

as treatment for anastomotic leak after ileal pouch-anal anastomosis: A pilot study. Techniques in Coloproctology. 2018;**22**(3):223-229

[80] Kochhar G, Shen B. Endoscopic fistulotomy in inflammatory bowel disease (with video). Gastrointestinal Endoscopy. 2018;**88**(1):87-94

[81] Lan NSB. Endoscopic fistulotomy vs. redo surgery for the treatment of pouch-to-pouch fistula in patients with inflammatory bowel disease. The American Journal of Gastroenterology. 2019;**114**:S535-S5S6

[82] Sze G, Khan F, Shen B. Combined endoscopic Fistulotomy and clipping for the treatment of fistula from the tip of the J-pouch to anastomosis. ACG Case Reports Journal. 2019;**6**(3):1-3

[83] Lan N, Hull TL, Shen B. Endoscopic sinusotomy versus redo surgery for the treatment of chronic pouch anastomotic sinus in ulcerative colitis patients. Gastrointestinal Endoscopy. 2019;**89**(1):144-156

[84] van Koperen PJ, van Berge Henegouwen MI, Rosman C, Bakker CM, Heres P, Slors JF, et al. The Dutch multicenter experience of the endo-sponge treatment for anastomotic leakage after colorectal surgery. Surgical Endoscopy. 2009;**23**(6):1379-1383

[85] Li Y, Shen B. Successful endoscopic needle knife therapy combined with topical doxycycline injection of chronic sinus at ileal pouch-anal anastomosis. Colorectal Disease. 2012;**14**(4):e197-e199

[86] Lian L, Geisler D, Shen B. Endoscopic needle knife treatment of chronic presacral sinus at the anastomosis at an ileal pouch-anal anastomosis. Endoscopy. 2010;**42**(Suppl. 2):E14

[87] Lan N, Shen B. Endoscopic treatment of Ileal pouch sinus. Inflammatory Bowel Diseases. 2018;**24**(7):1510-1519

[88] Lan N, Zhang L, Shen B. Post-index procedural gain in body mass index is associated with recurrent ileal pouch sinus after endoscopic or surgical therapy. Surgical Endoscopy. 2020;**34**(5):2127-2135

[89] Nyabanga CT, Shen B. Endoscopic treatment of bleeding diversion Pouchitis with high-concentration dextrose spray. ACG Case Reports Journal. 2017;**4**:e51

[90] Wu XR, Wong RCK, Shen B. Endoscopic needle-knife therapy for ileal pouch sinus: A novel approach for the surgical adverse event (with video). Gastrointestinal Endoscopy. 2013;**78**(6):875-885

[91] Khan F, Shen B. Inflammation and neoplasia of the pouch in inflammatory bowel disease. Current Gastroenterology Reports. 2019;**21**(4):10